9. 84

Juta's counselling handbook for healthcare professionals

Juta's counselling handbook for healthcare professionals

Robin Hamilton
Natalya Dinat

JUTA

Juta's counselling handbook for healthcare professionals

First published
Juta & Co.
Mercury Crescent
Wetton, 7780
Cape Town, South Africa

ISBN 10-digit: 0 7021 7275 8
ISBN 13-digit: 978 0 7021 7275 5

Typeset in 9 on 12 pt FphaseVagPierewiet

Project Manager: Melanie Wagner

Editor: Danya Ristic

Design and typesetting: Martingraphix

Cover design: WaterBerry cc

Cover photograph: Fiona Moosa

Printed in South Africa by Paarl Print,

22 Oosterland street, Paarl, South Africa

The baobab tree is highly regarded in Africa as it symbolises healing and protection. Baobab trees often serve as a meeting place for community discussions as well as for shelter, and its oils, leaves and fruits are used as medicine.

Contents

Acknowledgements

We gratefully acknowledge the assistance of the following people, who have made the development of this handbook possible:

Judith Ancer, Pierre Brouard, Professor Maeve Cougan, Dr Lionel Green-Thompson, Val Hunkin, Professor Christopher Szabo, Dr R Twycross, Jackie Williams and Dr Anne Wright.

About the authors

Robin Hamilton is a psychologist who has been involved in HIV/AIDS training on counselling and treatment issues for more than 10 years. He currently works for the Aurum Institute for Health Research in Johannesburg.

Natalya Dinat is an obstetrician-gynaecologist and palliative care specialist who teaches communication skills and palliative care at the Faculty of Health Sciences, University of the Witwatersrand.

Introduction

Origins of the handbook

The authors of this book, while working with faculty members at the University of the Witwatersrand, came to the realisation that providing healthcare professionals with sound clinical and medical knowledge is inadequate unless it is accompanied by training in basic communication and counselling skills. These generic skills do not apply only to particular situations, such as history taking and intake interviews. Rather, they can be utilised in a range of situations across the spectrum of health services, to:

- improve communication with patients
- help the health professional get across key messages to patients
- enable health professionals to have a more empathic understanding of the emotional dimensions of many medical issues
- improve patient adherence to medical regimens.

Hence it was decided that there was a need to develop basic counselling training. This handbook is a product of this decision. It can be used as a tool to train students in the health professions in a range of counselling skills. Moreover, it is hoped that the handbook will also provide a resource for practising these skills in clinical settings.

Principles

Certain principles underpin the approach taken in this book:

1. South Africa is a multicultural country, and it is important in providing counselling to be sensitive to context and difference. Differences are not merely most evident with regard to race and language, they are also to be found

in social class, gender, spiritual belief, political affiliation, sexual orientation, literacy and educational level. Throughout the handbook, cultural difference is illustrated, together with its possible impact on counselling.

2. Given the shortage in South Africa of qualified psychiatrists, psychologists, social workers, counsellors and other mental health professionals, often health care workers without specialist knowledge of counselling are called upon to perform a counselling role. It is hence important that as many health professionals as possible have some basic skills in counselling patients.
3. There is no one-size-fits-all solution for many of the issues discussed in this handbook. However, it is hoped that the handbook will sensitise readers to basic principles that may assist them in designing a counselling intervention that will be helpful to the patient and their family.

Using ordinary communication skills, taking history and providing information can be enhanced by making use of a counselling approach. The ability to use empathy, show respect and reflect feelings can be demonstrated in even the briefest interaction between health professional and patient. Communication and counselling skills can help to build a better relationship between health professional and patient, improve communication, ensure better adherence to treatment plans, and ultimately lead to superior health outcomes.

How to use this handbook

Structure of the handbook

The handbook comprises three parts:

1. The first section outlines some essential **principles of communication** that will be useful in most interactions between you as the health professional and your patient.
2. The second section describes basic generic **principles of counselling** which can be used in a wide range of situations. This section provides counselling theory and practical illustrations of how to apply the principles in everyday life. Hence the focus falls on the development and practice of skills. The section also suggests how to use counselling skills in brief interactions with patients (described as 'helping encounters').
3. The third section describes the application of **counselling skills to specific situations** in a medical setting. Examples include how to talk to patients about treatment options, how to give a patient and family members bad news, and how to conduct genetic counselling for prospective parents.

The emphasis in each section is on the practical application of theory. Each section also includes different kinds of boxed text:

- ❑ Sub-sections entitled **Tips** describe briefly how to deal with the issue under discussion.
- ❑ Sub-sections entitled **Pitfalls to avoid** highlight the most frequent errors made in dealing with the issue in question.

These sub-sections are designed to be read and assimilated quickly, so that you can apply the skills to practical situations.

Finally, some sections include examples of dialogue to illustrate the use of counselling skills in real-life settings.

Section A

Core communication skills

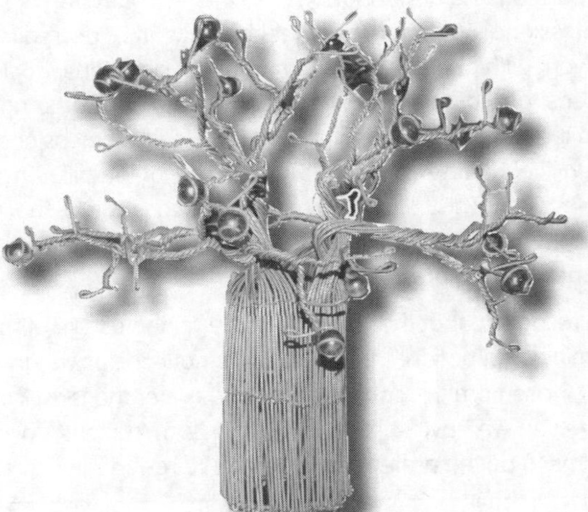

Note on terminology

Throughout the handbook we use the term 'health professional' to denote any healthcare worker accredited to work with patients, including dentists, dieticians, doctors, nurses, occupational therapists, opticians, physiotherapists and indeed anyone registered at the Health Professions Council of South Africa (HPCSA) or in one of the allied health professions. This includes those whose core competency is not counselling, that is, those who are not psychologists, counsellors or social workers.

We recognise that the current debate on the usage of the terminology 'patient' versus 'client' is not conclusive, and that those from the counselling world prefer the term 'client'. However, we have chosen to use the term 'patient' since it seems to be the preferred term of our target audience.

Overview of good communication skills

General principles of communication

Here are some general principles of communication that you may find helpful in talking to your patients:

1. Remember that every time you have contact with a patient, no matter how brief, you have the opportunity to convey a clear message.
2. If possible, try to focus ahead of time on what the key message or messages should be. Avoid trying to communicate too much detail, unless this is necessary. Detail can be confusing and detract from the key message.
3. Try to communicate only what is possible within the constraints of the setting. One key message well conveyed is better than five messages poorly communicated and not understood.
4. At the beginning, give the patient a rough idea of how long you can spend talking to them.
5. During any communication, be aware of the patient's feelings. Remember that it can sometimes be helpful to the patient just to reflect back to the patient their feelings, in the form of "You feel sad", "You feel worried", etc., and wait for the response.
6. Be aware of the limitations of the situation in terms of communication, for example:
   - ❑ language barriers between you and your patient
   - ❑ a noisy environment
   - ❑ lack of privacy – where other patients are also present
   - ❑ the patient is anxious or depressed (and so cannot take in much information)

- the patient's level of education
- the patient's intellectual capacity
- the patient's knowledge of Western medicine and healthcare
- what previous health professionals have told the patient.

7. If any of these limitations are present, try to adapt the communication to address the difficulty. For example, if language is a problem, use a translator (even a family member or another patient may be used to translate, if necessary, as long as issues of confidentiality are addressed); move to a quieter corner of the room or to the corridor, if the environment is too noisy; use accessible language if the patient has difficulty understanding, etc.
8. If you cannot address the difficulties with the patient yourself, try to refer the patient or at least give them some ideas of where to find help.

Understanding the importance of the patient

Remember that a patient is not just a number, a problem, a nuisance or an interruption of your work. A patient is the most important person in the hospital or clinic – the person who makes it possible for you to obtain training and earn a salary.

What do patients really want?

Patients appreciate the following:

- courtesy
- clean, comfortable surroundings
- professionalism
- genuine interest in their problems
- a clear explanation of what is happening to them
- empathy
- easy-to-read signs and instructions

- ❑ an assurance of quality
- ❑ knowing whom they are talking to
- ❑ a pleasant experience
- ❑ being attended to, or being told how long they will need to wait before they are attended to.

Patients dislike the following:

- ❑ rudeness and impatience
- ❑ hearing from a health professional: "But it's not my job!"
- ❑ broken promises
- ❑ a health professional taking a private phone call in the middle of a consultation
- ❑ prejudice and arguments
- ❑ jargon and difficult medical language
- ❑ being talked *about* by health professionals, rather than being talked *to*
- ❑ untidiness and lack of hygiene
- ❑ lack of punctuality
- ❑ lies and excuses for bad treatment
- ❑ red tape and excessive bureaucracy.

Tips for good communication

- ❑ Identify key messages in advance, if possible.
- ❑ Be realistic about how much you can communicate.
- ❑ Recognise the constraints of the setting.
- ❑ Reflect the patient's feelings.

Pitfalls to avoid

- ❑ Talking too fast.
- ❑ Using difficult words, technical terms and medical jargon.
- ❑ Trying to say too much.
- ❑ Being too abrupt.
- ❑ Failing to check the patient's language skills.

Information giving

One of the most common tasks of a health professional is to provide information on health issues to patients. There are various principles for providing such information. If you follow these principles, you are more likely to find that patients understand the information you give and are able to make better and healthier choices.

Providing information differs from counselling in that the focus is on conveying facts to the patient, rather than exploring their concerns and developing solutions. Nevertheless, there is still a need to develop a relationship with them in order to facilitate trust and to be able to check that the information is understood.

Understand whom you are talking to

You need to ascertain the most important characteristics of the patient or group of patients to whom you wish to give the information. Appropriate and effective questions to ask include:

- ❑ Does the patient speak or understand the language that you do? If so, how well does he or she understand this language? If not, what language does the patient speak? Do you need to use an interpreter? (See **Using an interpreter effectively** on page 23)
- ❑ Is the patient illiterate, partly literate or fully literate, and in which languages? (Remember that given the inadequacies of the South African education system in the past, even someone with a high school education may not be fully literate.) If the patient is not literate, using written materials to reinforce verbal messages is not helpful. Rather repeat the message in different words, or use simple drawings to reinforce your message.

- What are the social circumstances of the patient? For example, you would not tell an unemployed patient who is living in an informal settlement to buy vitamins or nutritional supplements.
- What understanding does the patient have of the ideas of disease and illness? You need to use the patient's language and frame of reference as much as possible in this regard.
- What is the patient's current understanding of the medical issue about which you wish to communicate?
- What are the patient's hopes and expectations of you? For example, does the patient expect you to provide a cure for the medical condition, and is this realistic or possible?

Remember that different patients may have very different needs in terms of information. For example, a female patient who has recently had a diagnosis of breast cancer will have a different need for information about cancer as compared to a female patient who has recently had a mastectomy.

Remember, too, that two patients diagnosed with the same illness – say a middle-class white housewife, and a rural African female farm-worker both diagnosed with cervical cancer – will have distinct needs based on their respective backgrounds.

Making assumptions about a patient can lead to poor or even harmful outcomes. A white farmer may be gay; Ms Dlamini may be a Buddhist and vegetarian. Don't make assumptions based on appearances!

Decide on key messages

Wherever possible, you need to decide ahead of time what the main messages are that you wish to convey to a patient or to a group of patients. Key messages should be reinforced by repeating them in various ways at different visits.

If you have enough time, start by giving the key messages in brief form and then expand on them one by one.

An example of key messages: Diet for people with hypertension

A health professional may need to talk to a hypertensive patient about a suitable diet. Three key messages regarding diet that might be selected are as follows:

1. reduce salt intake
2. reduce animal fats – red meat, butter, cream
3. reduce alcohol.

Consider providing information to a group

Think about whether it is possible to save time by providing health information to a group. Here are some relevant questions you can ask yourself:

- ❑ Is there a 'captive audience', for example patients with the same problem, all waiting in the same area to attend the same clinic?
- ❑ Do the patients share characteristics that will make it easier for you to communicate with them as a group? For example, are they of a similar age and do they speak the same language?
- ❑ Which messages can be communicated easily to a group? For example, the consequences of diabetics not taking insulin regularly.
- ❑ Are materials available to make communication more interesting? For example, TV and video equipment to show a video. If a video or film is shown, remember that on its own, this is a very passive form of communication. Follow up the use of such media by asking questions and encouraging a group discussion about the material, in order to get patients to take a more active role.
- ❑ Is the group of a reasonable size, that is, not larger than 16 people?

In a group discussion, ask one key question at a time, and encourage the group to discuss this. Questions should be pitched at a suitable level of understanding for the group.

Use every opportunity to talk to individual patients

You may be able to talk to an individual patient before, during or after a consultation. Even a few minutes can be used for simple health information provision. Give a small chunk of information at a time. It is useful to do this over a series of meetings with the patient, especially where the information is complex, for example triple-combination antiretroviral treatment for HIV-positive patients.

Check the patient's understanding

Always ask questions to check on understanding of key points.

A common error in asking questions is to say to a patient, "Do you understand what I have said to you?" Because of **social desirability**, most patients will provide the answer they think you want to hear, irrespective of whether or not they *have* understood. Hence they will most likely say, "Yes."

It is more useful to ask a patient, "Tell me what you understood, based on what I have just told you." Obviously this question takes more time to answer. However, it helps you to gain more accurate feedback about the patient's actual understanding.

Reinforce key messages

Make pamphlets available in a place where patients can help themselves to them, for example on a table outside a consultation room. It can be useful to hang posters on walls in an area where patients have to wait, and where they can read them easily.

Be sensitive to patients who are illiterate, or who have low literacy and cannot read written materials, including posters. For illiterate people, materials with a high proportion of illustrations may be helpful.

If there are community health workers in your area, consider working closely with them to reinforce key messages. Peer educators or school children working in health projects can also be effective.

Tips for effective information provision

- ❑ Think about the audience.
- ❑ Decide on key information messages.
- ❑ Convey health information in simple, clear language.
- ❑ Check that messages have been understood.
- ❑ Reinforce messages using posters, pamphlets and the help of community health workers.
- ❑ Consider using group presentations.
- ❑ Remember to reinforce health information in one-to-one interactions too.
- ❑ Give patients information materials to take away with them.

Pitfalls to avoid

- ❑ Communicating too much information at once.
- ❑ Not checking that the information is clear and focused.
- ❑ Not understanding the needs of the patient.
- ❑ Asking questions with high social desirability, such as "Do you understand?"

A theory of behaviour change

Introduction

Often in a health setting you will need to persuade a patient to change their behaviour because of undesired consequences in terms of health. Such efforts can cover a wide range of target behaviours, including:

- stopping smoking
- losing weight
- eating more healthily
- adopting an exercise programme
- practising safer sex to avoid contracting HIV/Aids
- taking medication regularly for a chronic condition such as hypertension or diabetes.

In encouraging behaviour change, remember to use the principles of counselling outlined in **Section B: Core counselling skills**, including:

- reflecting feelings and meaning
- asking relevant questions
- summarising
- developing a clear action plan.

Behaviour change is a complex process involving a wide range of factors. Ask yourself each of these questions when trying to get patients to change their behaviour:

- Is the individual concerned about good health?
- Does the individual perceive their vulnerability to risk as a result of the undesired behaviour?
- Do they believe that adopting the desired behaviour will reduce risk?
- Do they experience any unpleasant symptoms or consequences as a result of the undesired behaviour?
- Have they had personal contact with someone who has engaged in the undesired behaviour, and are experiencing negative consequences?

Behaviour does not depend on the individual alone. All behaviour takes place in a broader social context. Remember to take into account the individual's socio-cultural context, for example a young patient's attitude to condoms will be influenced by their friends' attitudes. Structural and environmental factors also play a role. For example, in the young person's cultural setting, is it seen as better to have sex 'spontaneously', without planning beforehand, thus making it more difficult to use condoms?

Reasons why patients resist change

- ❑ Fear of the unknown.
- ❑ Pace of proposed change is too quick for them.
- ❑ Change is not supported by the people around them.
- ❑ Change threatens existing networks,for example the patient's friendship circle.
- ❑ Denial of the need for change.
- ❑ Change goes against their core values.

Principles

Here are 10 key principles for helping a patient to change their behaviour:

1. Get the patient to recognise the need for change.

The first step in behaviour change is to get the person to acknowledge the need for the change. Without this, all effort at persuasion will be in vain.

Question to ask the patient: "Do you feel it is important to change this behaviour?"

2. Establish the patient's attitude towards the specific behaviour that needs to be changed.

A strongly positive attitude to behaviour change will be more likely to lead to the change.

A patient's attitude is affected by the subjective norms of those around them. Subjective norms are influenced by the beliefs of important reference groups or individuals in the person's life, and the desire to please those groups or individuals.

In some cases a person is more influenced by attitudes, for example an overweight older woman who wishes to lose weight and has a negative attitude about her body. In other cases a person is more influenced by the norms of their reference group, for example a young man whom you are trying to persuade to use condoms, but who feels condoms are not acceptable to his peers.

In each of these cases, the intervention to change behaviour will need to be different. With the older woman, it may be useful to focus on changing her beliefs about the difficulty of weight loss. In the case of the young man, it may be necessary to change his attitude toward condom use *and* to try to change the norms in his peer group.

Question to ask the patient: "How do you feel about the change?"

3. Be highly specific about the change in behaviour that you seek.

It is helpful for you to be specific about the behaviour change you seek. For example, just talking to the patient about 'exercising more' is not helpful, you would need to go into detail about the type of exercise that may be the most suitable, as well as when and where it should take place.

Each behaviour consists of four components: action, target, context and time. In the example given, the **action** regarding the exercise could be attending a gym, the **target** could be cardio-vascular exercise, the **context** could be exercising until the heart rate is elevated to 160 beats a minute, and the **time** could be four times a week for 20 minutes.

Remember that the factors associated with *starting* a new behaviour may be different to those required for *maintaining* the behaviour. For example, skills required for losing weight are different from those required for maintaining weight loss.

Question to ask the patient: "What exactly do you want to change?"

4. Encourage the patient to develop an intention to change their behaviour.

The stronger the patient's intention or commitment to do something, the greater the probability it will be done. The behaviour also requires opportunities and resources. If resources are not available, the best intention in the world will not help to achieve behaviour change. For example, wanting a patient to use condoms when condoms are not easily available or free is difficult.

Questions to ask the patient: "How motivated are you to change? Do you have the resources to change?"

5. Develop in the patient the belief that they have the ability to change their behaviour.

The belief in our ability to change behaviour is known as **self-efficacy**. A person with low self-efficacy will not believe they can easily change their behaviour, whereas a person with high self-efficacy will believe it is within their powers to do so.

You need to increase or reinforce a patient's sense of self-efficacy. One way of doing this is to make sure the patient has the necessary skills to carry out the behaviour, for example a woman who needs to take a particular medication exactly every 12 hours needs to have the skill to tell the time and a watch, or someone to remind her to do so.

Question to ask the patient: "Do you believe you can change?"

6. Help the patient to weigh up the benefits of changing behaviour against the disadvantages or obstacles. Help to perceive that the benefits outweigh the disadvantages.

People are more likely to change their behaviour if they perceive clear advantages or benefits from the new behaviour, for example an advantage of weight loss may be being able to fit into clothes of a smaller size, which the person could not wear previously.

One of the main reasons that people do not change their behaviour is that they perceive obstacles that will hinder or obstruct the behaviour, for example an obstacle to weight loss may be living with a family who likes to keep snacks in the fridge for consumption between meals.

It can be useful for the patient to make a list of benefits and obstacles. Help the patient to maximise the number of benefits, by suggesting any they may not have thought of. Then assist them to think of strategies to overcome the obstacles.

Questions to ask the patient: "What are the benefits of change? What are the difficulties or obstacles of change?"

7. Find out if the patient has an internal or an external locus of control. Adapt your strategy to fit this locus.

People are more likely to change behaviour if they perceive that they have an internal locus of control, that is, they feel they can exert control over events in their lives. By contrast, people with an external locus of control feel they are at the mercy of forces outside themselves, such as luck, chance, fate or other people. In this case, they are less likely to feel they can change their behaviour.

The political dispensation under apartheid contributed to many people feeling they had no control over their lives in South Africa. In addition, people who live in a traditional African culture or in other communally focused cultures are more likely to see the family, the group and the community as exerting more control than the individual.

In the case of a patient with an internal locus of control, strategies for change can be directed to the individual. In the case of a patient with an external locus of control, it may be useful to involve other family or community members in the change process.

Questions to ask the patient: "Do you feel you have control over change? Or do you think that it is in the hands of other people or fate?"

8. Help the patient to develop the skills to change their behaviour.

A patient who wishes to change behaviour needs to have various skills in order to translate intentions into action. Depending on the behaviour, these skills can include verbal communication skills, negotiation skills, assertiveness skills and problem-solving skills. Help the patient to develop these skills through role-play and through modelling the behaviour for them.

Question to ask the patient: "What do you need to learn in order to change the behaviour?"

9. Monitor the behaviour change.

The behaviour needs to be monitored to ensure that change actually takes place. Is the patient able to successfully carry out the new behaviour?

Question to ask the patient: "How will you know that the change has been successful?"

10. Develop strategies to reinforce and maintain the new behaviour.

It is crucial to reinforce the new behaviour, in order to ensure that it is maintained. Find reinforcement strategies which will ensure that the behaviour is repeated.

Question to ask the patient: "What will help you to carry on performing the new behaviour?"

An illustration of the model for changing behaviour: Weight loss

Step	Description	Practical example
1.	Get the patient to recognise the need to change their behaviour	Point out the problems with being overweight: risk of hypertension, diabetes, feeling less healthy, looking less attractive. Get the patient to acknowledge that this is linked to overeating
2.	Establish the patient's attitude towards the specific behaviour that needs to be changed	Ask the patient how they feel about going on a weight loss programme
3.	Be highly specific about the change in behaviour that you seek	In consultation with the patient, decide on an overall attainable goal, for example, to lose 20 kg and for their goal weight to be 75 kg
4.	Encourage the patient to develop an intention to change their behaviour	Help the patient to set more specific goals, for example to lose 2 kg per month using a combination of a diet programme and a light exercise programme

5.	Develop in the patient a belief that they have the ability to change their behaviour	Discuss with the patient whether they can visualise carrying out this programme. Ask them to make a list of personal strengths that can help them to lose weight
6.	Help the patient to compare the benefits of changing behaviour with the disadvantages or obstacles. Help them to perceive that the benefits outweigh the disadvantages	Make a list of the benefits of, and obstacles to, losing weight using the combination of diet and exercise. Discuss how to deal with the obstacles, such as finding transport to the gym
7.	Find out if the patient has an internal or an external locus of control. Adapt your strategy to fit this locus	If the patient has an external locus of control, invite family members or peers to join in the discussion about weight loss and get their support
8.	Help the patient to develop the skills to change their behaviour	Skills may include: • finding a diet plan • clarifying the terms of the diet plan with a dietician • clearing the house of unhealthy foods • practising how to shop for food differently • monitoring eating from day to day using a chart • developing a realistic exercise plan, with the help of a fitness consultant, for walking for 20 minutes three times a week.

		• talk to the patient about each of these aspects, or help them to identify who in their family or support system can help them to deal with each aspect
9.	Monitor the behaviour change	Keep daily records of both exercise and diet
10.	Develop strategies to reinforce and maintain the new behaviour	Think of social support, such as a friend to talk to when the urge to eat outside the diet is very strong. Think of rewards for following the new behaviours, such as an outing once a week, or buying a new item of clothing once a month

Having looked at this process in more detail, it should be clearer to you why just telling a patient what to do is usually not enough to change their behaviour.

Behaviour change is a complex process, involving many factors. However, the more factors you are able to address in talking to a patient about any prospective change, the greater the chance of lasting behaviour change taking place.

Tips for effective behaviour change

- ❑ Get the patient to recognise the need to change their behaviour.
- ❑ Find out the patient's attitude towards the specific behaviour that needs to be changed.
- ❑ Be highly specific about the change in behaviour that you seek.
- ❑ Encourage the individual to develop an intention to change their behaviour.
- ❑ Develop in the patient a belief that they *can* change their behaviour.
- ❑ Help the patient to compare the benefits of changing behaviour with the disadvantages or obstacles. Help them to see that the benefits are greater. Develop strategies for the obstacles.
- ❑ Find out if the patient has an internal or an external locus of control. Adapt your strategy to fit this locus.
- ❑ Help the patient to develop the skills to change their behaviour.
- ❑ Monitor the behaviour change.
- ❑ Develop strategies to reinforce and maintain the new behaviour.

Pitfalls to avoid

- ❑ Patient who needs to change doesn't see the need for change.
- ❑ Ignoring the social context.
- ❑ Having vague and unclear goals.
- ❑ Not having a clear plan for dealing with obstacles.
- ❑ Not using resources for change.
- ❑ Having no plan for maintaining the new behaviour.

Using an interpreter effectively

In a country like South Africa, the issue of what language needs to be spoken to facilitate communication is often a thorny issue. We have 11 official languages, and other languages may also need to be used, for example in dealing with patients from other parts of the world who live in South Africa, such as French-speakers from central Africa, Chinese immigrants or Shona-speakers from Zimbabwe. It is also important not to forget patients with hearing difficulties, who may need communication in sign language.

In many settings there may be a shortage of health professionals with proficiency in a range of languages. Hence it becomes necessary to use interpreters to communicate more effectively with patients who do not understand English.

Issue of confidentiality

The first issue that arises in using an interpreter is that of confidentiality. Whenever more than two people are present in a medical setting, there is a risk of confidentiality being breached. This issue needs to be discussed by the health professional with the potential interpreter *before* any translating is done.

If the interpreter is also a healthcare worker, for example a nurse translating for a health professional, professional ethics may already be in place to secure confidentiality. The same will not be true for other interpreters, such as a cleaner in the medical institution or a family member of the patient. In these cases, it is important to ask the interpreter to agree to treat the content of the conversation as completely confidential.

Remember that if a non-professional is acting as an interpreter, they may not be familiar with the concept of confidentiality. In this case it may be useful to spell out the concept in simple terms:

- 'Confidentiality' means not sharing with any other people anything communicated between the health professional and the patient.
- 'Other people' with whom information should not be shared include other health professionals and family members of the interpreter.
- The interpreter should also ensure that they do not disclose the identity of the patient to anyone else.

Effective translation

Here are some principles for effective use of interpreters:

1. Recognise that having an interpreter present alters the relationship between you and your patient, as there is now a third person involved, who brings in their own perspective.
2. Remember that for interpretation to work, the interpreter needs to be competent in both the source and the target languages.
3. You should try to spend time before meeting the patient in briefing the interpreter on their role. Emphasise translating accurately, word for word, not changing meaning or adding detail.
4. Remember that interpreting doubles the time it takes to communicate any message. So try to communicate more simply.
5. Communicate one point at a time. Ask only one question at a time. Asking more than one question is likely to confuse both interpreter and patient.
6. Avoid using technical terms or medical jargon, which will be difficult to translate.
7. Give the interpreter time to think about how best to translate both into the language of the patient, and back into your language.

8. Be aware of the most common errors that can occur in translation:
   a) Because of embarrassment the translator leaves out sensitive information, such as when the client talks about sex.
   b) The translator adds information not given by the patient.
   c) The translator condenses the information provided by the patient and so leaves out crucial details.
   d) The interpreter takes over the interview, replacing some or all of your questions with their own.
9. Address the patient and not the interpreter. Observe the nonverbal language of the patient carefully when using an interpreter. It can give you an indication as to whether all the verbal messages of the patient are being translated by the interpreter.

Tips for using an interpreter

- ❑ Where possible, brief the interpreter before meeting the patient.
- ❑ Ensure that issues of confidentiality are addressed.
- ❑ Talk more slowly and say less.
- ❑ Communicate only one point at a time.
- ❑ Avoid complex messages and medical jargon.

Pitfalls to avoid

- ❑ Using a friend or relative of the patient for translation, and not checking that the patient is comfortable with this.
- ❑ Speaking too fast.
- ❑ Trying to say too much.
- ❑ Using complex and difficult language.

Power dynamics in medical settings

As a health professional, you need to be aware of the power dynamics that operate in a medical setting. In any clinic or social service setting:

- patients have less power than health professionals
- patients must conform to the times and systems of the clinic
- patients must abide by the clinic's rules
- patients must rely on you for information and resources
- patients have no control over access to information.

Other power dynamics that may affect interactions between you and your patients include differences in:

- economic and social class
- gender
- age
- levels of education and literacy
- home language
- race
- sexual orientation.

The difference in power often leaves the patient feeling very vulnerable, and creates an environment where they feel less comfortable in talking about personal issues. For example, an adolescent girl may feel very uncomfortable about talking to an older male doctor. In the same way, an illiterate black farm-worker may feel uncomfortable in talking to a black urbanised female nurse. Even though both farm-worker and nurse may be black and use the same home language, the differences in terms of gender, social class and education may still create difficulties.

Patients tend to imbue health professionals with great power. A patient may expect you to take control, to be all knowing and all powerful, and to offer the perfect cure. In turn, patients may see themselves as ignorant, helpless and passive.

This power dynamic can be tempting for the health professional. Being seen as the 'great expert' seems flattering. However, the flip side is that the patient feels powerless and does not take responsibility for their health and treatment. This pattern makes communication difficult. The patient's expectations of you are often unrealistic. Disappointment is likely to result, in turn leading to non-compliance with treatment and not returning for follow-up visits.

For these reasons, it is helpful to be aware of the power dynamics between you and your patient. Always try to address the power dynamics wherever possible.

Tips for reducing the effects of power dynamics

- ❑ Introduce yourself by name.
- ❑ Greet the patient politely and make sure you understand their name correctly. If you are unsure, ask the patient.
- ❑ Try to avoid additional barriers that will make the patient more anxious, for example a desk between you and them.
- ❑ Talk about your relationship with the patient being a partnership. More importantly, try to make it a genuine partnership.
- ❑ Treat patients' concerns seriously.
- ❑ Ask patients for their ideas on particular issues.
- ❑ Avoid medical jargon and difficult terminology. Translate what you say into the patient's type of language.
- ❑ Don't assume understanding or knowledge.
- ❑ From the beginning, take the time to explain disease and treatment to patients. It will save time in terms of getting better compliance with treatment regimens and reducing defaulting from treatment.
- ❑ Be aware of differences between you and the patient. Be open and honest with the patient about these. Ask the patient's help in bridging the divide.
- ❑ Do not be afraid to say, "I don't know" when you do not know the answer to a particular question.

Pitfalls to avoid

- ❑ Ignoring differences between you and the patient.
- ❑ Labelling a patient as stupid or ignorant.
- ❑ Failing to take the time to build a relationship.

Errors in communication

Common errors

At some point every healthcare professional finds themselves communicating poorly, making one or more of the errors below. It is helpful to realise that nobody can entirely avoid these communication errors.

Criticising

Criticising means making a negative evaluation of a patient, their actions or attitudes. Some health professionals believe that they ought to be critical of patients' actions or attitudes, or these will never improve. However, constant criticism will eventually lead a patient to feeling incompetent and will diminish their self-esteem.

Example: "You drink too much and then get into fights – you've got nobody but yourself to blame for your problem."

Name-calling and labelling

'Name-calling' refers to putting down or stereotyping a patient by calling them foolish, lazy, nagging, clumsy, etc. These labels prevent you from getting to know the real person and often describe only one aspect of the person.

Example: "You must be really stupid if you can't remember when your next appointment is."

Praising evaluatively

Praising evaluatively means making positive judgements of a patient's behaviour as a gimmick to manipulate the patient to do as you wish. It also creates anxiety and guilt when the patient realises they can't perform well all the time.

Example: "You're such a clever boy. I'm sure you will always take all your pills."

Ordering

An order is a solution sent coercively and backed by force. When coercion is used patients typically feel resistant and resentful. They may deliberately do the opposite to assert themselves. Patients who are constantly given orders may become very compliant and submissive. They start to believe that their ability to make their own decisions is unsound and this tends to undermine their self-esteem too.

Example: "Stop smoking right now."

Threatening

A threat is a solution sent with an emphasis on the punishment that will follow if the solution is not implemented. It usually fails to work, and encourages patients to lie to cover up their behaviour.

Example: "You'd better start eating now or we'll feed you through tubes up your nose."

Moralising

Moralising occurs when solutions are backed up with the force of social, moral or religious authority. It fosters anxiety in the patient, arouses resentment, tends to thwart honest self-expression and invites pretence. Typically, words like 'should' and 'ought' are used.

Example: "As a Christian woman you should always be faithful to your husband."

Excessive or inappropriate questioning

Excessive questions can kill communication. The patient being questioned may feel interrogated and harassed and become defensive. The other common error with questioning is to use too many closed questions that usually require only a 'yes' or 'no' response, and are frequently unhelpful because they elicit little useful information.

Example: "Do you know all about Aids?"

Glib advice

Glib advice is often an insult to a patient's intelligence, as it implies a lack of confidence in the capacity of the person to understand and cope with their problem. Another difficulty is that the adviser seldom understands the full implications of the problem.

Example: "You must go home now and tell your family that you are pregnant."

Diverting

This involves changing the topic so that the health professional switches to their own concerns. You may divert for many reasons. You may want the attention focused on yourself, be uncomfortable with the emotions stimulated by the conversation, or you may simply lack the skill to listen.

Example: "Speaking of headaches, I had a terrible one yesterday."

Logical argument

Logical argument involves attempting to convince the patient with an appeal to facts or logic, without considering the emotional issues involved. When a person is in distress, their feelings are the main issue. It is very frustrating when someone tries to talk a patient out of feeling something by telling them how illogical they are being.

Example: "There's no need to feel worried about the operation. Only 2% of patients don't survive."

Glib reassurance

Reassuring means trying to stop the patient experiencing negative emotions. Glib reassurance *seems* to be a way of comforting a person but it actually does the opposite. It can be a form of emotional withdrawal on the part of the health professional. It is also used by people who like the idea of being helpful but don't like the emotional demand that goes with it.

Example: "Don't worry about the results of your HIV test. Everything will be fine."

Tips for avoiding communication errors

- ❑ Every person is prone to some particular communication errors. It is useful for you to become aware of what your communication errors are. You need to notice when you resort to these.
- ❑ Often, a health professional resorts to a communication error when tired or unable to think about how to respond to a patient. Try to avoid communication errors wherever possible.
- ❑ It is helpful to show real interest in the patient. This means listening before drawing any conclusions, and putting aside preconceptions or stereotypes that you may have about 'this sort of patient'.
- ❑ It is important for you to try to understand the patient's unique situation. Remember that no patient is exactly like any other.
- ❑ Try to express real empathy, and imagine what it would be like to be in the patient's shoes.
- ❑ The patient needs to be encouraged to develop competence and motivation to solve their own problems.
- ❑ Cultivate the ability to be silent when silence is needed. Sometimes silence can be more emotionally healing and helpful to the patient than even the wisest words.

Section B

Core counselling skills

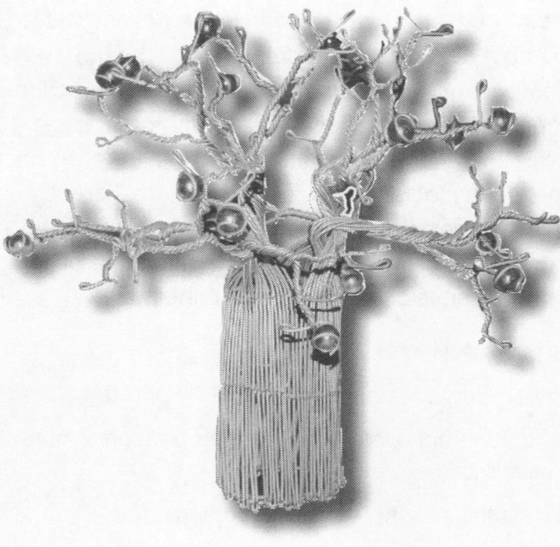

Counselling and psychotherapy

Defining counselling

Counselling has been defined by Alta van Dyk (2005) as a process in which you, working within the framework of a special helping relationship, use specific skills to assist patients in dealing with their problems. Note that you, as the health professional, are not responsible for *solving* their problems.

In essence, counselling is a person-centred approach in which the counsellor aims to *listen* to the patient and to help *solve certain problems* in the patient's life. The most essential core component is taking the time to listen to the patient. For many patients, especially those from poorer socio-economic backgrounds, being listened to and really heard is an experience that they have not had before. Sometimes the experience of being listened to by itself – without necessarily even moving on to focusing on and solving the problem – provides a sense of genuine relief to the patient.

Aims of counselling

Counselling can be seen as having three primary aims:

1. To help the patient to manage their problems more effectively.
2. To help the patient to develop coping skills.
3. To empower the patient to become more effective in the future at helping themselves.

Differences between counselling and psychotherapy

In practising counselling, it is helpful for you to be aware of the scope of counselling and its limitations. Counselling is *not* the same as psychotherapy, and you need to keep the distinction in mind. Some of the important differences are as follows:

- Counselling may be practised by people from a wide range of professions and by laypeople who do not necessarily have a formal background in psychology. Lay counselling training is usually of limited duration, and most often lasts 5–10 days.
- In contrast, psychotherapy is usually practised by professionals with a specific qualification in psychology or psychiatry. Their training extends over a number of years.
- Counsellors are not trained to deal with mental illness, whereas psychotherapists are equipped to do so.
- The focus of counselling is on addressing short-term problems. It is solution focused. Counselling is usually of limited duration – sometimes only a single session, or, more rarely, up to 10 sessions.
- Psychotherapy may be also short term, or it may be provided over months or even years. Psychotherapy may seek to address a wider range of problems, including underlying personality issues, childhood issues and emotional trauma.
- The practice of psychotherapy is governed by professional regulations and determined by professional boards. In contrast, counselling in South Africa currently has no formal regulation, although moves toward the creation of more formal structures are being made.

Limits of counselling

It is important for you to recognise the limitations of the skills you possess, and to understand when and where to refer your patients to other professionals for help.

The following issues lie outside the scope of counselling, and are therefore inappropriate areas in which to intervene. You should not counsel a patient who:

- is suffering from severe mental illness, including psychosis, major depression and bipolar disorder
- is seriously suicidal
- has personality disorders, including antisocial personality disorder, narcissistic personality disorder and borderline personality disorder
- has severe intellectual impairment.

In all these situations it is advisable to refer the patient to a suitable professional who can help, for example to a psychologist, a psychiatrist, a psychiatric nurse or a social worker.

Brief counselling encounters

In South African medical contexts, it is sometimes not possible to provide formal counselling. The burden on public hospitals often limits the time that you can spend with a patient. Pressure to see many patients in a day and the lack of privacy make it almost impossible to engage in a formal counselling process that may take 40 minutes or longer and extend over many sessions.

However, this does not mean that the counselling process cannot be useful to you. The principles of counselling can be helpful for even the shortest encounter. Because of the practical constraints, it is probably more accurate to talk of **brief counselling encounters** than counselling sessions. In the box over the page are some pointers for how to be effective in even the most limited health professional–patient contact.

Tips for brief counselling encounters

- ❑ Privacy is often difficult. But make a plan to attain it.
- ❑ If you are in an open clinic, try to make the counselling encounter more private: sit with the patient in a corner apart from other patients and staff.
- ❑ If you are seeing the patient in a multiple-bed ward, close the curtains around the bed, sit close to the patient and talk in a low voice.
- ❑ Show respect and address the patient by name.
- ❑ There is no need for formal contracting. Explain you are here to listen to the patient and how much time you have to talk.
- ❑ Focus on talking less and listening more.
- ❑ Reflect the patient's feelings: "You feel … ".
- ❑ There is no time to find formal solutions. If time allows, one or two suggestions on how to deal with the problem may be helpful.
- ❑ Point your patient toward useful resources.
- ❑ Remember that listening for even five minutes can be helpful for someone to whom nobody really listens at all.

Ethics of counselling

All healthcare professions have ethics. So too does counselling. In medical ethics Hippocrates' notion of doing no harm is an important guiding principle. In counselling, too, it is important at the very least to avoid doing any harm to the patient.

Health professionals' values and ethics have an important part to play in determining the success of the helping process. The most important values underlying the process are respect, empathy, congruence, empowerment, confidentiality and working with difference.

Respect

Respect means treating every individual in counselling with the same positive regard. It means not judging the individual. An important distinction in counselling is to distinguish between the patient and their behaviour. While you may find yourself disapproving of a patient's behaviour – for example, having unprotected sex – this needs to be separated from your acceptance of the patient as a person. Respect needs to be given to the patient irrespective of their behaviour.

Empathy

Empathy means trying to see the world from the patient's perspective – you try to imagine being in the patient's shoes. This is not always easy to achieve, for example where the patient has very different values or a different cultural background to yours. However, it is essential if a sound health professional–patient relationship is to be built.

Empathy involves acknowledging human diversity and avoiding stereotyping people. It means recognising that each individual is unique and different to any other person. Effective empathy means accepting that your values are not better, just different from the patient's values.

Congruence

Congruence or genuineness means that you are real, honest and sincere as much as possible. It means too that you avoid playing a role or using a façade. You should try to steer away from patronising or condescending to the patient. It is also important that you not over-emphasise the helping role.

Empowerment

Empowerment is a significant value in counselling. You try to empower the patient to take responsibility for themselves, and to use creatively whatever resources are available in the patient's environment. Your attitude is that the patient has the resources to benefit from the counselling process and to live their life more effectively. Underlying this value is a belief in the patient's ability to grow and change. In order to empower the patient, it is important that you resist the urge to 'rescue' the patient. Rescuing encourages dependency and gives an implicit message that the patient is not able to take responsibility for themselves.

Confidentiality

Confidentiality means that you keep to yourself whatever you and your patient discuss in the counselling session. It is important to maintain confidentiality in order to help the patient to feel safe and to trust you enough to talk freely, without censoring their thoughts or feelings. If they do not feel safe, they may fail to disclose important information. In turn, the counselling relationship may become superficial and distant.

Preserving confidentiality entails a range of measures. These include taking steps to make sure that:

- ❑ the counselling room or space is reasonably soundproof
- ❑ files containing confidential information are not left lying around for others to see

- you do not gossip about the patient to other health professionals, or discuss patients with people outside a professional setting.

Sometimes you may need to share the information that the patient discusses with you in counselling with other health professionals in order for you to provide better care for the patient. Here, you must make the need to share information clear to your patient, and obtain their permission before you share it. If the reasons for sharing information are made clear, most patients will happily grant consent.

The only situation in which confidentiality can be broken without the consent of the patient is in the case of the patient saying anything to indicate they may be a risk to themselves or to someone else, that is, in the case of the patient being suicidal or homicidal. Here, you have a higher ethical responsibility, which is to protect life, and you may disclose information to others to ensure the safety of the patient or those around them.

Working with difference

In South Africa there is a wide range of differences in patients, including race, gender, socio-economic class, religious belief or lack thereof, level of literacy, political belief, sexual orientation, degree of urbanisation, language, nationality, age, intellectual ability and attitude to Western medicine. These differences, especially culture, have been used in the past to divide South Africans and create a sense of 'them and us'. It is useful to have some tools to work with cultural difference, as provided in the box below.

Tips for working with cultural difference

- ❑ Remember that in any encounter between two people, culture plays a role. You and your patient will never be identical in terms of the cultural influences on both of you.
- ❑ Never assume that people from the same cultural background as you think the way you do. There are often subtle differences.
- ❑ If you often encounter people from a particular culture in your work, try to find out about them.
- ❑ Never forget there are probably multiple cultural influences on your patient. Ask about all of them. Don't just make assumptions based on the most visible differences, such as gender and race.
- ❑ If you are having difficulty with a patient because of big cultural differences, find someone from the same culture as your patient to help bridge the gap. For example, if you are an urbanised young white man counselling an elderly rural Zulu-speaking woman, and you have difficulty communicating, enlist the help of an urbanised Zulu-speaking nurse to help you to communicate.
- ❑ Remember that culture is never static and unchanging. The way in which people practise their culture changes over time.
- ❑ Respect people's cultural beliefs, even if you do not agree with them. Respect will always secure better communication from patients.
- ❑ Be curious about other people's cultures. Ask questions sensitively.

Developing self-awareness

Developing self-awareness is a crucial aspect of becoming a better health professional. The more you know about yourself, the more effectively you will be able to use your personality in counselling. Knowing yourself also means becoming aware of your personal values and norms. In this way you can start to learn about your 'blind spots', that is, the issues you feel strongly about, where your emotions can get in the way of a rational and considered response to the patient. For example, many people have a powerful emotional response to the idea of child sexual abuse. So when you encounter children who have been sexually abused – or perhaps even an adult abuser – it can be easy for your emotions to cloud your judgement.

You can help yourself to develop greater self-awareness in the following ways:

- Get in touch with your feelings and responses to situations.
- Notice where you are most able to empathise and where you struggle to do so. This can alert you to your values. Where do your biases and prejudices make communication difficult? Everyone has areas of difficulty. What is most helpful is to acknowledge these areas and be conscious of them.
- Notice your style of non-verbal communication. How do you use or not use your arms and hands when you talk? What tone of voice do you use?
- Ask a close friend or colleague for feedback on your personal style. Ask them to tell you what it is about your style that makes it easy for others to engage with you, and what makes it more difficult. Try to alter the difficult characteristics, such as an unfriendly tone of voice, or not making eye contact.

- Notice where your personal issues can make counselling difficult. For example, having had a loud, bossy parent may make it hard for you to empathise when a patient is loud and demanding. If a personal issue gets in the way of effective counselling, consider talking to a counsellor yourself about it.
- Supervision and mentoring can also help you to develop greater self-awareness. See the section below on these two issues.

A generic counselling model

There is no single, universal method for practising counselling. Nevertheless, in South Africa the ideas of Egan (1998) and Van Dyk (2005) have provided a useful model for lay counselling. This model can be practically adapted for a wide range of cultural contexts, which is often necessary in South Africa. The model outlines a four-phase process. It will be described in more detail below.

Basic counselling model

The basic steps in the counselling model are as follows:

1. Build rapport.
2. Encourage the patient to tell their story.
3. Develop a deeper understanding of the problem.
4. Decide on what action to take.

It is important to note that counselling is not a strictly linear process. In practice, the phases outlined here overlap and interact. Skills used in one phase may be useful in other phases too. The model is just a guiding **framework**, particularly useful for health professionals who are learning these skills for the first time, for anyone who finds that the process has 'got stuck', and for reviewing the counselling process after it has been completed. This is not a rigid model, yet it can provide a useful structure for each counselling session.

The model is applicable to a setting where more formal counselling takes place. In practice, health professionals are likely to have brief counselling encounters (see **Brief counselling encounters** on page 36 for more details).

Phase I: Building rapport

The goal of phase I is to establish an open and trusting relationship with the patient. Achieving a good relationship will enable the patient to feel safe and comfortable enough to talk about personal issues and to disclose information to you.

An important first step is for you to introduce yourself to the patient. Then you should form a contract with the patient clearly, in order to define the objectives, limits and process of counselling (see **Contracting** below for more details of this process). The process of contracting should take place at the beginning of the counselling session, and need not take more than a few minutes.

The physical setting in which counselling takes place can also help to establish trust. Wherever possible, it should include the following components:

- ❑ a private room, where you and the patient will not be interrupted or overheard
- ❑ two chairs facing each other, or at a slight angle to each other, without an obstacle such as a desk between them
- ❑ comfortable lighting, a reasonable temperature, ventilation and tissues.

The constraints of medical settings mean that these criteria cannot always be met. For example, it may be necessary to counsel a bedridden patient in a ward where other patients are present. Here, privacy may best be provided by drawing curtains around the patient's bed, and you moving closer than usual to the patient and speaking in a softer but still audible voice, so that your conversation cannot be overheard by other patients in the ward.

When the physical setting for counselling is less than ideal, you need to make whatever arrangements are possible to secure privacy and a comfortable space, and to prevent interruption.

Skills in phase I

Important skills for you to utilise in phase I include the following:

- **Using attending skills** (see **Attending** below for details).
- **Showing empathy and respect**. From the first contact the relationship needs to be built on your sincere attempt to see the situation from the patient's perspective. Respect means treating every patient the same.
- **Using listening skills**. You need to listen carefully to the patient, and to look out for the following aspects: the patient's experience (what has happened), the patient's behaviour (what the patient has done or has failed to do), the patient's feelings (how the patient feels in relation to their experiences, especially the problem itself) and your own feelings (how the patient impacts on you).
- **Tracking non-verbal behaviour**. This refers to all the physical cues that the patient uses to communicate, and includes posture, gestures and eye contact. Are the non-verbal behaviours of the patient aligned with what they are saying, that is, do they qualify what the person is saying, or do they contradict the words the patient is using?
- **Following the patient**. You should let the patient take the lead in talking, at least initially, and not impose an agenda of your own.
- **Responding to the emotional tone of the patient's story**. It is helpful to reflect the feelings of the patient by using phrases like "You feel … ", followed by a feeling word. This is important in establishing a close bond between you and the patient, and communicating empathy. Sometimes just acknowledging their feelings, and not doing anything more, is sufficient to help a patient.

Phase 2: Encouraging the patient to tell their story

The second phase has as its primary goal to get the patient to tell their story in order for you to get a better understanding of the situation. The focus here is on gathering information to get a broad perspective of the current situation, as well as what the patient would prefer the situation to be. You need to be genuinely curious and wanting to learn more, especially about the patient's behaviour, experience, feelings and thoughts.

You should use the following guidelines in this stage:

- Learn and use the patient's own vocabulary and means of expression, as this communicates understanding and empathy.
- Ask questions about the patient's context, for example the patient's family, support system and home environment.
- Avoid making suggestions about solutions and do not give advice, even though this may be very tempting.
- Revisit issues in order to gain a better understanding, if necessary.
- Focus on the process of developing the problem or difficulty over time.

Skills in phase 2

The following skills are very useful in phase 2:

- **Linking feelings to content** (see below for more details).
- **Identifying specific feelings, experiences and behaviour**. It helps to focus on specific experiences that the patient has had, and to avoid vague and unclear generalisations.
- **Using minimal verbal responses** such as 'mmm' and 'uh-huh' to communicate to the patient that you are listening intently.

- **Using open rather than closed questions** to probe for more information (see below for more details).
- **Being more accurate in terms of empathy,** that is, reflecting feelings and content more effectively.

Phase 3: Developing a deeper understanding

The goal of phase 3 is for you and the patient both to gain a better understanding of the problem situation. If the patient's story has been well explored in phase 2, it will be possible to gain a better understanding in phase 3 by asking questions judiciously and thoughtfully. You start to build up an understanding of the problem and to share your understanding with the patient.

Skills in phase 3

The types of skills that are useful in phase 3 include:

- **Advanced empathy**. This means not just reflecting what the patient has said, but also trying to 'read between the lines' to what the patient may be hinting at.
- **Clarifying**. This refers to using simple language to mirror back to patient what they have said, to help the patient to see the situation more clearly, and to confirm understanding.
- **Summarising,** which means condensing what the patient has said into a couple of sentences. It helps both you and the patient to identify the key issues.
- **Partialising,** which refers to breaking the problem down into smaller, more manageable parts.
- **Giving clear feedback or challenging**. This is a difficult skill to practise. Essentially it involves dealing with discrepancies or contradictions in the patient's story, for example between different aspects of what is said, or between what is said and how it is said. It is important that this is done empathically and without judgement, to maintain your relationship with the patient.

- **Staying in the here-and-now**. Counselling which focuses on the present is more effective. It means examining the current status and impact of the problem. It also means looking at how the patient comes across in the session. And it is very helpful to acknowledge what is happening right now. For example, if a patient talks about a particular problem and begins to cry, it is important to reflect this, for example, by saying, "I can see the situation makes you feel really sad".

Phase 4: Deciding on what action to take

The goal of phase 4 is to explore options for action and to make a decision on the best intervention to make. It is important to distinguish between you offering advice or providing a solution, and you and the patient deciding together on the best option to take. The idea here is to avoid imposing advice or a solution on the patient, which is often not followed if it is your opinion only.

Skills in phase 4

The problem-solving model of phase 4 has six steps (see **Partialising and problem-solving** below for more details):

1. Defining the problem.
2. Brainstorming solutions.
3. Weighing up alternative solutions.
4. Choosing the best solution.
5. Developing an action plan.
6. Taking action.

If the patient returns for a follow-up visit, or if you see the patient again, it is possible to review the action that was taken, or examine why it was not taken or if it failed. If the solution was not entirely successful, the process can be re-examined. Phase 4 can be worked through again to find further solutions.

Some patients find it extremely difficult to come up with solutions themselves. This may be because they have an external locus of control – they tend to see themselves as being at the mercy of other people, fate or events they have no control over. They do not think they can exert any influence over what happens to them. In contrast, people with an internal locus of control feel they can influence events, direct the course of their lives and make things happen. If a patient has an external locus of control, they may need more help from you in the form of suggestions about possible solutions. Here you must be more proactive and sometimes even directive.

Contracting

In the first phase of the counselling process, the process of contracting is essential to facilitate the success of the counselling session. It takes only a few minutes to do this, but helps to ensure that there is agreement between you and the patient about the framework within which the process will take place. Without a clear contract, there is a much greater chance of misunderstanding and miscommunication.

Contracting needs to cover all of these issues:

1. **What is counselling?** In South Africa, given the limited resources for mental healthcare, many people will not have had experience of counselling. This fact makes it necessary to explain in simple terms what counselling involves. A suggested explanation would be: "You and I are going to spend some time talking together about … [the issue or problem]. This will help us to understand it better and think of ways to deal with it".
2. **How long will the counselling process take?** The length of time required may be difficult to define before counselling begins, but you need to give the patient a rough idea of how long you intend to talk to them initially – perhaps 20 to 30 minutes. If you do not define the time required, the patient may expect counselling to be a brief process taking only 5–10 minutes, and may be impatient to leave once this time has passed.
3. **Confidentiality**. Assuring confidentiality is important for the development of trust and openness. You should define for the patient what confidentiality means. One way to express this is: "What is said between us stays between us, and is not shared with others without you being consulted first".

4. **Collaboration**. You should tell the patient that counselling involves a collaborative relationship, which means that both parties work together, and the patient is given full opportunity to talk. This contrasts with many health professional–patient relationships, where the health professional does most, or all, of the talking.
5. **What will be discussed?** It is useful to decide, before the counselling process begins, what the key issue in counselling will be. The issue may change as counselling proceeds, and further discussion between you and the patient will then be necessary to renegotiate the issue under consideration.
6. **Agreement.** Does the patient understand the issues discussed, and is the patient willing to agree to these conditions? If not, you should discuss any difficulties the patient may have with the process before proceeding further. Once agreement is reached, the counselling process may proceed.

Examples of contracts

A formal contract

"Mrs S, can you and I spend some time talking together about your cancer and the problems it is causing you? It will help us to understand the problems better and decide together what we should do about them.

We have 30 minutes to talk. We are just going to talk about the cancer now, not your pension problem.

"What is said between us here stays between us, and I won't share it with other people without consulting you first. Are you okay about this?"

An informal contract

"Mr M, we have 10 minutes to talk about your STI. Is that okay?"

Listening and attending

Listening

Listening involves your ability to comprehend the messages that the patient conveys as they tell their story, and includes both spoken and non-verbal components.

According to Egan (1998), listening includes the following key skills:

- ❑ Listen to and understand the patient's **verbal (spoken) messages**. Listen for the patient's mix of experiences, behaviour and feelings.
- ❑ Listen for the patient's **non-verbal messages**, conveyed through posture, body movement, gestures, facial expressions, tone and pitch of voice, pauses, silences, blushing, breathing, grooming, dress and physical appearance.
- ❑ Listen for the **context** of the patient. In what social context does the patient live, and what effects does this have on them? Listen for the *whole* context of the patient's messages, and not for isolated details.
- ❑ Listen always using **empathy**. You should put aside your own perspective. Listen for what it is like to live in the patient's world.

Attending

Attending means using physical and psychological means to let the patient know you are 'with' them. Using effective attending skills helps the patient to feel you really care about them, and opens the door to the patient talking freely about their problem.

The acronym SOLER is often used to summarise basic attending skills, and represents the following concepts:

- **S** stands for **sit squarely**. This means you should sit opposite the patient, facing them. If facing the person squarely is experienced as too threatening, a more angled position may be used. However, there should be no physical barriers between you and the patient, such as a desk or a table.
- **O** stands for **adopt an open posture**. You should avoid crossed arms and crossed legs, which can communicate not being available or not being open to the patient.
- **L** stands for **lean forward** towards the patient. But leaning needs to done sensitively – if it occurs too early in the counselling relationship, or is too extreme, it can be experienced by the patient as anxiety provoking. A slight inclination towards the patient is better for communicating empathic listening.
- **E** stands for **make appropriate eye contact**. Making eye contact communicates to the patient that you are interested in what they have to say. But be aware of cultural differences – see **Cultural sensitivity** below for more details.
- **R** stands for **relax**. You should try to relax and be natural. Fidgeting should be avoided.

Cultural sensitivity

In a multicultural country such as South Africa, attending skills need to be applied with cultural sensitivity. For example, in rural African culture too much eye contact can be experienced as rude or confrontational. It can also be regarded as rude for a younger person to make eye contact with an older one. It may be regarded as more respectful for a younger person to look away when addressing an older person. You need to observe the patient and see what form of eye contact is most comfortable for them.

The distance that you sit apart from the patient may also be different in different cultures. You should not sit too close or too far away. Take your cue for a comfortable distance from the patient.

You need to be familiar with traditional forms of greeting, and make sure to pronounce and spell the patient's name correctly. In some cultures, addressing an older person requires a more formal approach, and you may find it possible to develop a better relationship if you avoid using first names, which can suggest over-familiarity. If in doubt, ask the patient how they would like to be addressed, rather than trying to guess.

Reflection

Reflection is useful in every stage of the counselling process. Reflection involves you mirroring back to the patient what you have heard the patient saying. The reflection has two components: **reflecting meaning** and **reflecting feelings**. You need to be able to listen at both levels to reflect effectively. By reflecting both meaning and feelings, you create a climate of understanding and trust, which enables the patient to feel safe enough to share more and to explore the issue more deeply. It also gives the patient permission to have these feelings.

Reflecting meaning

Reflecting meaning is also known as **paraphrasing**. It involves you listening carefully to what the patient is saying and then saying back to patient what you hear.

For example:

Patient: Since I started chemotherapy, I feel so tired, and it's all the time. I don't have any energy to cook or clean. I can't keep up with the housework. It's so hard. I just can't do all the chores I have to do every day. Everything is going to pieces.

Nurse: I hear you say that since you started treatment, you're so tired, and you can't keep up with your chores any more.

Reflecting feelings

You should respond to the patient's feelings by identifying the correct class of emotions. Most health professionals identify five main classes of emotion, corresponding to:

- **happy** feelings – joyous, pleased, delighted, thrilled
- **sad** feelings – depressed, forlorn, abandoned, devastated
- **angry** feelings – irritated, resentful, furious
- **unhappy** feelings – confused, bored, guilt-stricken, worthless
- **fearful** feelings – scared, worried, terrified.

Once a feeling has been identified, the next step is to identify the correct intensity of emotion. For example, fear may vary in intensity from *concerned* to *fearful* to *worried* to *terrified*.

Some patients – especially men – feel uncomfortable in talking about feelings. It may be helpful for you to focus initially on experience and behaviour, and only later introduce and name specific feelings. Men may also feel more comfortable in being asked to describe their physical (bodily) responses to particular situations.

It is important to remember that patients do not always express their feelings verbally. You need to note non-verbal cues to feelings, such as posture and facial expression. It is also helpful to note which feelings a patient is less comfortable expressing, and to reflect this too. For example, a woman may be socialised not to express anger easily.

For example:

Patient: I can't believe it; yesterday I was well and now you tell me that I only have another six months to live. How is it possible? How can I cope? It's too much for me to handle.

Nurse: You feel shocked and scared …

Tips about reflecting feelings

- ❑ Having feelings or emotions is one of the core experiences of being human. All of us feel validated if someone else shows they recognise our feelings.
- ❑ Getting in touch with the patient's feelings is perhaps the most important aspect of counselling.
- ❑ Reflecting feelings serves a number of purposes. It helps the patient to feel understood and acknowledged. It is deeply confirming and validating. It communicates empathy and caring. It builds a good relationship between you and the patient.

- If you do nothing more than just reflect the patient's feelings accurately, you will have assisted the patient. Sometimes this is all there is time for, and it is helpful in itself.
- Most health professionals initially find reflecting feelings the hardest of all the tasks of counselling. It takes practice. At first, it may feel very formulaic to say, "You feel …" to the patient. Later it is easier to find an individual and comfortable way of doing this.
- Women find it easier to talk about feelings than men do, especially about vulnerable feelings. Men often find it easier to talk about how a situation affects them and so will refer to feelings indirectly.
- There are also cultural differences. Some languages, such as English, have many words for the expression of feelings. Other languages, such as Zulu, have relatively few words, and use metaphors. So people often use other expressions for feelings, such as "It is a very heavy thing I have to carry" to express feeling overburdened.
- You should not fear inaccurate reflection of feelings. If the reflection is correct, the patient will acknowledge it. If your reflection is wrong, the patient will usually correct you. However, even an inaccurate attempt to reflect will communicate your empathy for the patient's situation.

Linking feelings to content

Linking feelings to content has this basic formula:

"You feel [name the relevant emotion] … because [name the relevant situations or experiences which give rise to the feelings] ..."

An example of this would be: "You feel devastated because you have been told this week you can't have a heart transplant."

The reflection of feelings and linking the feelings to particular content is important throughout the counselling process. It is an important way in which you can express empathy, and it offers support to the patient and creates a context in which you can intervene more effectively.

It is important for you to avoid:

- using clichés in reflecting feeling, such as "I know how you feel"
- merely repeating parrot fashion what the patient has just said
- giving no response at all, especially to very emotionally loaded content; here 'yes', 'mmm' and 'I see' are better than giving no response at all (but see the section on **Use of silence** below).

Advanced reflection of feelings

At a later stage in the counselling process, it may be helpful for you to use more advanced empathy to explore new themes and feelings. You should then listen for the following (Van Dyk, 2005):

- What is the patient only half-saying?
- What is the patient saying in a confused way?
- What is the patient hinting at?
- What is the message hidden in what the patient is saying?

Advanced reflection should still try to connect the patient's feelings with an event or behaviour.

However, a word of *caution* is needed here: advanced reflection of feelings still focuses on what the patient is actually trying to say, not on your interpretation of what the patient is saying. Advanced reflection of feelings can then achieve the following goals, by helping the patient to:

- make explicit what has only been implied
- see themes in their stories
- make connections between different stories
- propose educated guesses about what is happening to them
- see the bigger picture.

This is an advanced skill that you can acquire with time and practice.

Use of silence

It is natural for newly trained health professionals initially to feel uncomfortable with silence during the counselling session. However, it is important for you to develop the skill to judge the quality of the silence.

A silence can be comfortable, and it can be a time for the patient to reflect on what has been said, and to gather their thoughts together to decide what to say next. In this situation, words from you might be experienced as awkward or intrusive.

However, there are other kinds of silence where the lack of response from you to the patient's words can be experienced as unhelpful. If trust has not been established between you, a non-therapeutic silence could be interpreted as you struggling to find something to say, or you being judgemental or non-accepting of the patient.

With time and experience, it is possible for you to develop sensitivity to the nature of a silence and the best response in those circumstances.

Clarifying

In phases 3 and 4 of the counselling process, it is important for you to clarify what the patient is saying, using the techniques of probing and asking questions.

Probing

Probing entails you using questions, statements and short comments to help the patient to explore important issues in greater detail. Probing can take many forms, including using questions, making requests for more information, repeating a phrase or a few words in a questioning manner, or using non-verbal communication to encourage the patient to think further about an issue.

Asking questions

You need to be careful in asking the patient questions. It can be easy for too many questions, asked one after another, to come across to the patient as if they were an interrogation. You need to question sparingly, and ask only the most essential ones.

You should avoid asking too many closed questions. Closed questions are questions that often begin with the words 'is', 'do' and 'have', for example "Have you accepted that you have diabetes?" They tend to have short answers, sometimes just 'yes' or 'no'. They usually elicit less interesting information from the patient. There is a place for closed questions, but they generally tend to make the patient say less rather than more.

You should instead focus on asking open-ended questions, which require more than a simple yes or no or short answer. Open-ended questions often start with 'how', 'what' or 'tell me about', for example "Tell me how you feel about being diabetic". They are usually experienced by the patient as less threatening and encourage more complex, fuller descriptions of problems.

It is better to avoid asking the question 'why' too often. Although it is an open-ended question, it is often difficult for the patient to answer and can sound interrogatory.

You should also avoid asking leading questions, where the patient can tell the answer you expect from them, for example "Have you taken all your pills?" Patients tend to respond to these questions in the way they think you desire, and so you learn very little from them. A better question here would be: "Tell me what it has been like for you taking your pills".

In a brief counselling encounter open questions may not be possible because of time constraints. Here closed questions may be more useful for eliciting simple information quickly.

Summarising

In phases 2, 3 and 4 of the counselling session it may be useful for you to summarise what has been said. A summary serves two major purposes: it helps both the patient and you to obtain clarity about the major themes of counselling, and it gives the patient an opportunity to move on to other issues.

Summaries can be useful at different times in the counselling session:

- At the beginning of a second or successive counselling session, a summary can give direction when a patient is confused about where to start, and can prevent the patient from talking about the issues that had already been discussed in the previous session. Summarising here can help the patient to move on to new issues.
- When a counselling session seems to be lacking direction or to be stuck, a good summary on your part can help the patient to focus on the relevant issues.
- When it is time to introduce a new phase in the counselling process, a summary is often a useful starting point.
- At the end of a counselling session, it is also useful for you to summarise the work of the session.
- Even at the end of a brief counselling encounter, it may be useful to summarise quickly and to suggest a way forward.

Appropriate challenging

Initially you will need to establish a good rapport with the patient. Once this goal is achieved, it is possible to explore the issue that the patient has brought to counselling in more detail. One of the skills that is useful in phase 3 of the counselling model and beyond is the use of appropriate challenging.

Challenging needs to be used sensitively. The timing is crucial – earlier on in the counselling process, the patient will not respond well to challenges. Later, the trust that has been established makes it possible for you to engage in feedback or challenging. Challenging can focus on any of the following:

- ❑ A discrepancy between what has been said and how it has been said, for example a patient talks about his mother dying, but smiles as he talks about the loss.
- ❑ Inconsistency between different statements made by the patient, for example the patient talks about having first tried to fall pregnant a year ago, but later mentions she has wanted to fall pregnant for three years.
- ❑ A discrepancy between what the patient has said and what you believe to be true.

However you need to carefully consider the wording of a challenge in order to avoid it sounding like a criticism. For example, a challenge in the first example given above might be: "You have just told me about your mother dying, and yet as you spoke about it, you smiled. I wonder what that is about ..."

Partialising and problem-solving

In phases 3 and 4 of the counselling process, partialising and problem-solving will be useful skills.

Partialising

Partialising means breaking down a problem into parts. Partialising is particularly useful when a problem appears to be large and overwhelming, with no immediately apparent solution. By breaking down the problem into its components, the task of finding solutions is made easier, because the smaller problems will then each be easier to solve.

Problem-solving

You should make use of problem-solving only once phase 4 of the counselling process has been reached. It is less helpful to engage in problem-solving earlier, before you and the patient have attained a full understanding of the situation. The problem-solving model involves six steps:

1. **Defining the problem**. Having proceeded through phases 1 to 3 of the counselling process, it should be relatively easy to define the core problem. It is useful to define the problem in terms of specific needs.
2. **Brainstorming solutions**. Encourage the patient to think of as many solutions as possible to the problem. Write all of them down, no matter how silly or crazy they may seem. You should add your ideas only when the patient has been able to suggest some first.
3. **Weighing up alternative solutions**. Here the patient and you draw up a list of pros and cons for all suggested solutions. The solutions are then compared.

4. **Choosing the best solution**. Usually the best solution is the one with the fewest disadvantages and the most advantages. The patient should be encouraged to make the choice – remember that they will have to implement and live with the consequences of the solution.
5. **Developing an action plan**. Draw up a practical plan together of how to implement the solution. Include specifics such as what, when, where and how it will be done.
6. **Taking action.** The patient may feel anxious or afraid of taking action, especially if the change appears to be difficult. You should help the patient to explore the benefits, and suggest possible forms of support for taking action.

If the patient returns for a follow-up visit, it may be possible for you to re-evaluate the action that was taken, or examine why the action was not taken, or, if it failed, why it did not work. If the solution was not entirely successful, the process can be re-examined and a new plan of action can be developed. Phase 4 can be worked through again to find further solutions.

Reviewing, referring and terminating

Reviewing

Toward the end of the counselling session, it may be useful for you to engage in a process of reviewing the session together with your patient. Useful questions for this feedback process include the following:

- What can the patient take away from the session that was useful?
- What about the session was less useful?
- What did the patient learn from the session?
- Is there any unfinished business, that is, are there issues that were not adequately dealt with during the session? Can these issues be carried over to a further session, or do they need to be dealt with outside the formal counselling process?

It can be helpful for you to summarise what was accomplished in the session, and to check that the patient is in agreement with this understanding.

The review process is useful for the patient. However, it can also help you to reflect on your performance, and to adapt ways of working in future sessions with the same patient or with other patients.

Making referrals

At some point you are likely to come across a patient whose needs fall outside your area of expertise. It is a responsible action for you to admit that you are unlikely to be able to help and to explain the situation to the patient. Ideally, you should try to refer your patient to another person who can offer specialist help.

First you should gather information about the patient and carefully consider who could be an appropriate referral. If necessary, you should contact individuals or organisations to find out if they are an appropriate referral. Any details about the patient should be kept confidential.

You may be able to explain to the patient the limits to the help you can offer in the same conversation in which you also offer the patient some suggestions about people or organisations that are likely to be better able to help. Sometimes, you may need to gather ideas to bring to the next session.

It is the patient's choice as to whether to accept your suggestions. But you also need to be honest when the patient does not have a choice about whether or not they can continue talking with you.

Depending on the circumstances, you might offer names and telephone numbers for the patient to make direct contact. Sometimes it may be more appropriate to introduce the patient personally or to write a letter of referral.

You can also continue to have informal contact with the patient and to support them in a general way. It is always helpful to check that the referral was useful, since the patient may appreciate other suggestions if the first suggestion has not worked.

Terminating a counselling session

It will often be evident to both you and the patient when the time has come to terminate a counselling session. So it may not always be necessary to terminate a session formally. However, a number of termination tasks need to be addressed in order for termination to be complete:

- It is useful to repeat the plan of action that was agreed upon in the session, and to clarify what you and the patient will do before the next counselling session.
- In the case of the patient needing to be referred elsewhere for further help, it may be advantageous to clarify how the referral will take place.
- It is important to decide whether a follow-up session needs to be held, and, if so, to arrange the date and time.

Health professionals often feel uncomfortable about bringing the session to a close. However, continuing the counselling session beyond its natural end-point conveys a message to the patient that they are not capable of dealing with life alone, but need you to prop them up. Termination, in contrast, sends a message of confidence that the patient is capable of continuing alone with the work begun in the session.

Terminating the counselling process

In a formal counselling session the action of terminating the counselling process can occur for a number of reasons. Termination can take place because the patient's presenting problem has been resolved or is no longer a problem. It may occur because you decide counselling can be of no further benefit to the patient. It can also take place because you both decide by mutual consent not to continue, or the patient needs to be referred elsewhere for specialist help.

If the patient and you have seen each other for a number of sessions, it is best to prepare the patient for termination before the last session. Wherever possible, try to avoid announcing termination and terminating in the same counselling session.

Preparation for termination will involve the following tasks:

- Discussing the patient's possible emotional response to the idea of termination. Feelings evoked may include sadness, anxiety, fear, relief, calm, and even resentment or anger at you for 'abandoning' the patient.
- Reflecting on the complete process of counselling, and what has been achieved.
- Acknowledging the issues that have not yet been resolved, and how these could be dealt with after the sessions have ended.
- Discussing how the patient will continue on their own the work begun in counselling, once the sessions have ended.
- Allowing the patient to acknowledge your contribution, where relevant.
- Recognising the emotional challenges of ending for both the patient and yourself.

In a less formal counselling encounter, terminating will focus on three points only:

1. Alerting the patient to the fact that only a few minutes are left of the counselling session.
2. Summarising in a sentence what was talked about.
3. Mentioning what the patient should do next.

Support and supervision

Informal support

Ideally any healthcare setting has a positive network of informal support between colleagues. Often health professionals:

- share ideas with each other, within the bounds of confidentiality with regard to patients
- pass on useful information about contacts and helpful resources
- look out for colleagues who appear overloaded, puzzled or distressed
- support each other so that everyone is more able to support the patients.

Being busy makes this less easy to carry out. You may be subject to an unrealistic workload that leaves no time for reflection and exchange of ideas. It is hard to ask for or accept help from colleagues if the culture of the healthcare setting does not tolerate admission of doubt or mistakes.

Supervision

Regular supervision is especially important for people who use counselling skills within their job:

- to ensure that the work is consistent with the values and objectives of the overall organisation – this kind of supervision can be crucial when health professionals are dispersed between sites or shifts and do not regularly meet each other
- to provide personal support for health professionals – helping services of any sort make considerable demands on people's energy and creativity.

Supervision is needed by everyone, not just by newly qualified health professionals and not only when there is a problem. There should never be a sense that supervision is only for those people who cannot cope.

Health professionals need to retain the humble knowledge that they can also benefit from help, rather than feeling that they always have to be the ones who do the helping.

It is important to talk about work with a colleague within the appropriate boundaries of confidentiality. It may be helpful to use that person as a sounding board. Health professionals who do not have an opportunity to talk within supervision will either keep all their concerns to themselves or may be tempted to talk with friends or family, which raises further issues about breaching confidentiality.

In supervision it is helpful to talk through the difficulties or uncertainties of counselling. A good supervisor should also call the person's attention to what they have done well and competently.

Good supervision draws on communication and counselling skills, although there are differences between supervision and working with a patient. Supervisors have an obligation to ensure that your work is consistent with the values of the organisation, is productive and is ethical. So supervisors may sometimes be more directive than you can be with a patient.

Section C

Counselling skills for specific situations

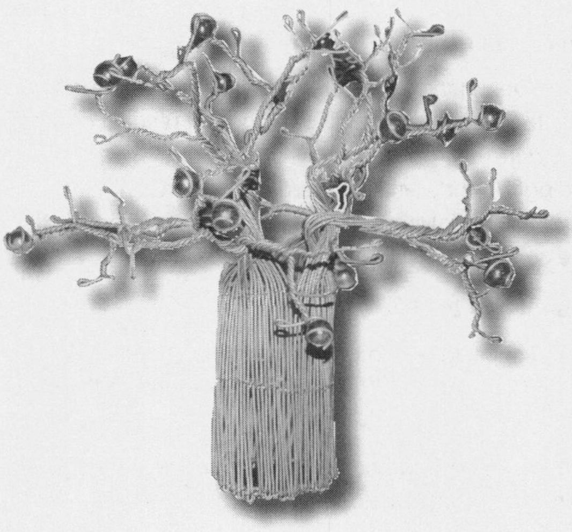

Obtaining informed consent

Introduction

Health care has undergone a shift away from the paternalistic approach, where the health professional was considered the expert who could make decisions about people and treatment, toward a more equal approach, in which the patient's point of view is respected and taken into account. The principle of respect for the autonomy of the individual now requires health professionals to help patients to make their own decisions free from pressure.

Remember, in the process of obtaining consent you need to utilise the ethical principles of empathy, respect and patient empowerment. Counselling techniques such as contracting, building rapport, reflecting feelings and meaning, clarifying and problem-solving are all useful here too (see **Section B: Core counselling skills**)

Consent and the law

The patient's right to informed consent is protected in the South African Constitution of 1996. The Bill of Rights in the Constitution (1996) says:

> Everyone has the right to bodily and psychological integrity, which includes the right –
>
> a) to make decisions concerning reproduction
> b) to security in and control of their body
> c) not to be subjected to medical or scientific experiments without their informed consent.

The Constitution also says:

> Everyone has the right to have access to –
>
> a) health care services, including reproductive health care.

The National Health Act, 2003 deals specifically with consent, and also refers to the right to refuse consent to health services. A number of legal cases in common law have helped make clearer what the law expects of health professionals. This is outlined below.

Not obtaining informed consent for any procedure or treatment can lay you open to legal charges, as well as a case before the HPCSA.

What does the patient need to know?

According to McQuoid-Mason (2006), the patient needs to have both knowledge and an appreciation or understanding of:

- the nature of the condition or disease they are suffering from
- the range of diagnostic procedures and treatment options available
- the benefits, risks costs and consequences associated with each option
- the right to refuse, and an explanation of the implication, risks and obligations of such a refusal.

Patients often struggle to understand highly technical medical language. It is very important, when providing the patient with all the relevant information, that you avoid medical jargon and difficult terminology. If medical terms need to be used, explain them to the patient in layperson's terms. Use language that is accessible to the patient.

Benefits of informed consent

Informed consent brings a number of important benefits for both you and the patient:

- The patient may feel less anxious because they know and understand what is being done to them.

Remember that fear of the unknown is a major stress trigger for many patients.

- ❑ The patient is likely to be more co-operative in the treatment and intervention.
- ❑ The patient feels respected and included, which is good for the health professional-patient relationship.
- ❑ You feel clearer about the patient's commitment to the treatment or intervention.
- ❑ The process of obtaining informed consent allows any misunderstandings to be cleared up earlier.
- ❑ Informed consent promotes the patient's sense of ownership of the treatment plan and is likely to lead to more committed health-promoting behaviour.

Implicit and explicit consent

There are two major types of consent: implicit or implied consent and explicit consent. **Implied consent** occurs when, for example, you ask the patient to roll up their sleeve for blood to be drawn, and the patient does so. There is no clear verbal discussion about the action – the patient's consent is implied by their co-operation.

In contrast, there is a move toward **explicit consent**, especially for major procedures or interventions, for example, any form of surgery. Here you talk to the patient about the intervention, allow them to ask questions, and then obtain verbal or, better still, written consent for the intervention.

People from different cultural and non-Western backgrounds may feel more comfortable making a decision about informed consent in consultation with family members or significant others. It may be helpful to a patient to ask if they need to consult anyone else or if anyone else needs to be included in making the decision for consent. If others need to be involved, the patient could be given written material to take away and read, or the others could be invited to come along to the next appointment with the health professional.

Written consent is now preferred for all major procedures. If the patient is literate, give them time to read the consent form and to ask questions. If the patient has limited literacy or is illiterate, read the form out loudly and slowly, and then allow time for discussion and questions.

An illiterate patient cannot sign a form, but they can provide a thumb-print as evidence of consent. It is then useful for someone besides yourself to sign as evidence of witnessing the thumb-print.

Children and consent

The Constitution defines a 'child' as a person under 18 years of age. The National Health Act, 2003 states that users of health services have the right to participate in any decision affecting their personal health or treatment. This right extends to children who are sufficiently mature enough to understand the effect and nature of the health service, even though they may not have the legal capacity to consent.

Children under the age of 18 may not consent or refuse consent to an operation unless it is a termination of pregnancy (TOP). An 'operation' is defined as 'any form of surgical procedure major enough to require an anaesthesia'. 'Treatment' is defined as 'cae, in terms of medication, nursing and any other therapy, designed to cure a disorder'. Although the children must be consulted, if mature enough, the parent or guardian must give consent to the operation.

Children under the age of 18, but over the age of 14, may however give or refuse consent to other medical treatment without the assistance of their parent or guardian. Thus, for example, a nurse may dispense contraceptives to a teenager older than 14 years.

Female children of any age may consent or refuse consent to a TOP, provided they have the capacity to understand the nature and effect of the procedure.

A new Children's Act has been passed but is not yet in practice. It is expected that the new act will only be implemented in 2008. When it is implemented, it will allow any child over 12 years of age to consent to medical treatment without the parent or legal guardian's permission being required.

You may feel trapped when you counsel a child and their parent or guardian about the need for treatment, and the child wants the treatment but the parent or guardian does not. The law makes it clear that your primary responsibility is to the child. In this situation, try to talk the matter through calmly and slowly with the parent or guardian, listening to all their concerns – this most often resolves the difficulty.

Remember, however, that even if the parent or guardian continues to refuse treatment, the child still has the right to the treatment. If the situation cannot be resolved, consult somebody in higher authority.

Exceptions to informed consent

The only exceptions to informed consent are:

- medical emergencies
- testing a patient for HIV after a needle-stick injury; if the patient refuses to be tested, their blood can still be drawn, but the patient should not be informed of the result
- patients with cognitive impairment
- mentally ill patients (Aids Law Project, 2005).

Even in medical emergencies any information known about the patient should still be taken into account before treatment is provided. For example, a person known to be a Jehovah's Witness should not be given a blood transfusion.

Mentally ill patients or patients with cognitive impairment usually cannot give informed consent, in which case consent should be sought from the next of kin, if at all possible.

Tips for informed consent

- ❑ Explain the procedure or intervention in simple, non-medical language that the patient can understand.
- ❑ Explain the benefits and risks of the intervention.
- ❑ Discuss alternative interventions and their risks and benefits.
- ❑ Ask the patient to paraphrase the discussion, and clarify any misconceptions.
- ❑ Let the patient make up their own mind.
- ❑ Get consent in writing, where practical and necessary.

Pitfalls to avoid

- ❑ Using medical jargon.
- ❑ Pressurising the patient to make a decision.
- ❑ Ignoring family members, when the patient wants to involve them in helping to make the decision.

Stopping smoking

Most people who smoke find that smoking is an addiction that is very difficult to stop. Just telling a patient to stop smoking is not sufficient to get them to do this. It is preferable to formulate a detailed plan with the patient, using the principles of behaviour change. See the principles listed in **A theory of behaviour change** on page 13, and take the points listed below into consideration as well.

Help the patient to research their habit

Suggest to the smoker that prior to giving up smoking, they thoroughly research the issue in the following ways:

- Compile a list of **trigger situations** that make the smoker more likely to light up, for example having a drink or a cup of coffee, feeling down or depressed, feeling happy, boredom.
- Make a **plan** of how else to deal with each of the trigger situations, for example take a walk if feeling depressed.
- Think of all the **negative effects** of smoking, for example heart and lung disease, cancer, strokes, halitosis, high cost, social disapproval.
- Make a list of the **benefits of giving up**, for example breathing more easily, no unpleasant taste in the mouth in the morning, reduced risk of disease, greater quality of life, longer lifespan.
- Plan an **alternative rewarding** use for the money spent previously on cigarettes or tobacco.

Make a plan for stopping

Beforehand, it is crucial to develop a clear plan with the patient for stopping smoking. Without this plan efforts to stop usually fail. Impulsively stopping 'cold turkey' works for a few smokers only.

The patient should be encouraged to fix a target date to stop smoking. The individual should finalise a clear plan about how to deal with trigger situations, such as having a cup of coffee after a meal. Before the planned date for stopping approaches, the smoker can choose to take one of three strategies: gradually cut down on the number of cigarettes smoked per day, change to a less preferred brand, or continue smoking as usual. It is important in this period to encourage the smoker to visualise a life without smoking.

If the patient can afford it, you should discuss using one of the following options to support the act of giving up smoking:

- hypnotherapy
- acupuncture
- nicotine replacement therapy – in the form of nicotine patches, gum or nasal spray
- Smokenders or a similar course for stoping smoking
- taking the drug buproprion (Zyban).

Provide ideas for support

Support from other people in making a major life change such as stopping smoking is vital for its success. You can suggest sources of support such as:

- ex-smokers who have quit successfully
- family members and friends who wish to encourage the patient to stop
- another patient or a friend who wishes to stop smoking at the same time
- phoning the Stop Smoking helpline for support (011 720 3145); helpful booklets are available in English, isiZulu and other languages.

Giving up

Warn the smoker that the most difficult period is likely to be the three days following giving up. During this period physical withdrawal symptoms are very uncomfortable, and can include dry mouth, postnasal drip, bronchitis, headache, nausea, irritability, restlessness and insomnia. The patient should be advised to try to drink plenty of water, take moderate exercise, keep busy and have healthy snacks on hand.

Resisting returning to smoking

A challenge for smokers who try to give up the habit is that psychological dependence is hard to break. It is hence important to encourage the ex-smoker to find healthy behaviour patterns that can replace the habit of smoking. Here are some suggestions:

- Having worry beads or a bracelet to occupy the hands is soothing for some people; others like to play with a pencil or a small object.
- Chewing gum or brushing teeth often is useful for some ex-smokers. Other people find the oral stimulation of sipping a glass of water soothing.
- Doing gentle exercise or going for a walk when the urge to smoke arises.
- Cleaning the home or engaging in other physical work is distracting for some, as is taking up a new hobby or home improvement project.
- Making a plan for how to spend the money saved by not smoking.

Other useful ideas for resisting the temptation to smoke again include the following:

- Staying away from friends and acquaintances who smoke.
- Avoiding social situations where smoking is acceptable, for example bars and shebeens.

- Thinking of only having to cope with not smoking for one day at a time.
- Keeping a glass jar of used cigarette butts close by. The appearance and smell of the butts can serve as a powerful deterrent when the impulse to smoke arises.
- When temptation arises, reading a list of diseases linked to smoking.
- Not attempting to make any other major life changes at the same time as giving up smoking.

Establishing a new life without smoking

For most smokers, six months without smoking is an important turning point. The focus becomes how to maintain the new behaviour. However, warn the ex-smoker that even once smoking has stopped, the urge to start again will never completely disappear. It is important to be constantly vigilant, and also to find ways of rewarding the commitment not to smoke.

Tips for giving up smoking

- Encourage the patient to research the habit thoroughly before stopping.
- Suggest strategies for trigger situations.
- Get the patient to visualise life without smoking.
- Encourage social support.
- If possible, use strategies such as medication, support groups and stop-smoking programmes.
- Prepare the patient for withdrawal symptoms.
- Suggest that the patient develop a plan to avoid returning to smoking.

Pitfalls to avoid

- Stopping 'cold turkey'.
- Forgetting to reward the new behaviour.
- Failing to get support from others for stopping.
- Getting into situations that encourage smoking.

Communicating bad news

Health professionals are often expected to communicate bad news about health to patients and their family members. Bad news can be defined as any information about the patient's health that is likely to negatively and dramatically change their view of their future. It includes:

- progressive life-threatening illness with no cure, such as terminal cancer
- a threat to the patient's physical or mental health, for example a diagnosis of bipolar disorder or severe heart disease
- a limitation of the patient's quality of life, for example a diabetic patient needs to have a lower leg amputated
- news of the death of a relative, for example parents hearing that their child died during an operation.

You may well find breaking bad news to patients and their family members distressing. It goes against the primary purpose of health professionals – to heal and cure illness. It often elicits a negative reaction from those who receive the bad news, including anger and denial, which may make you uncomfortable.

Few health professionals feel they are equipped with the necessary interpersonal skills to tell bad news tactfully. And few health professionals have the resources to deal afterwards with their own feelings and reactions to having had to communicate unwelcome messages.

Counselling skills such as empathy, respect, reflecting feelings, summarising, questioning and appropriate use of silence can be extremely useful in breaking bad news to both patients and their families (see **Section B: Core counselling skills**).

Wherever possible, break up giving bad news into two separate sessions: in the first session, give the news and support the patient through the emotional reaction; and in the second session, help the patient to plan practically what to do. But sometimes two sessions may not be possible, and you may need to do all of this in one session.

Tips for breaking bad news to patients

- The news needs to be communicated slowly enough so that the patient has time to get used to it. If told too abruptly, the patient may go into a state of shock and denial.
- Be alert to cues from the patient expressing concern about their condition, for example questions, or hints that the situation is not good. This may signal how ready the patient is to hear the news.
- Choose an appropriate time to do it: when there is enough time to talk, when there is as much privacy as possible, when the patient and you will not be disturbed. Be familiar with the details.
- Check first how much the patient knows about their condition.
- Then make a clear statement such as: "I am concerned that this may be more serious than we thought".
- Pause to allow the patient to take in the fact that serious news will follow.
- Give the bad news in small chunks. Allow time between statements for the patient to take it in. Allow silence, if necessary.
- Allow time for questions, and answer them honestly to the best of your ability.
- Reflect feelings appropriately. All emotional reactions are normal, and can include anger, shock, denial, sadness, fear and calm. There can also be no apparent reaction, which often indicates shock.
- Stay connected to the patient through touch and eye contact where appropriate.

- ❑ Avoid giving unrealistic reassurances.
- ❑ Give some realistic hope. Even when an illness is terminal, mention treatment options to reduce pain or help to maintain human dignity.
- ❑ If the patient asks how long they have to live, give a prognosis of either 'days', 'months' or 'years'. This is more appropriate than giving a specific figure, such as months.

Talk to the patient again later. Check their level of understanding. If the patient goes into denial, this needs to be respected. Denial may be a useful coping mechanism. Do not insist that the patient has to see things the way that you do. Patients have as much right not to know as they have a right to know about their health.

Tips for breaking bad news to family members

- ❑ It is usually preferable to communicate bad news separately to the patient, and to the partner or family members.
- ❑ Some family members may be more prepared to hear bad news about the patient than others.
- ❑ Try to talk to family members together, if possible, to make sure they are all given the same news in the same way.
- ❑ It is better to talk first to adult family members, without the presence of children, and to communicate to children later, or to encourage the adult family members to talk to them.
- ❑ Give information in small, manageable chunks.
- ❑ Allow time for questions. Give written contact details for questions that may arise later.
- ❑ Be realistic about treatment options, and do not offer false hope.
- ❑ Accept that family members may react with a wide range of emotions, including anger, blame, sadness and denial.
- ❑ Family members may cope by blaming you. Do not take such blame personally.

Avoiding collusion

Try to avoid collusion, such as in the case of some family members requesting you to withhold bad news from other family members or from the patient. Remember that your primary concern is the patient's best interests, not the family's best interests.

If you collude with the family, often the result will be stilted communication, more lies, tension and increased isolation of someone, usually the patient. The collusion may cause unfinished business and block the grieving process later.

If family members ask you to collude, acknowledge how difficult the situation is for them. Acknowledge that they *think* this is the best solution. However, also tell them this does not mean it *is* the best option.

Try to get permission from the family members to find out about what the patient understands and wants to know about their condition. This will allow you to talk to the patient, and break the news if necessary.

Pitfalls to avoid in giving bad news

- Using complex medical jargon.
- Giving the bad news too quickly.
- Dropping the bombshell and then just leaving the patient or family alone.
- Avoiding giving answers to uncomfortable questions or using vague language.
- Offering unrealistic reassurance.
- Giving bad news in a setting that provides no privacy.

Talking about sexuality

Normalise sex

Because of the strong influence of social conservatism and religious faith, South Africans have a long tradition of not discussing sex and sexuality openly. The prevailing attitude was that sex should not be talked about. Despite a more liberal legal framework, today this attitude still holds true in many communities.

Thus one of the most important interventions you can make is to normalise sex for the patient. This means talking about sex frankly and without embarrassment. It also involves saying to the patient that sexual feelings are normal. Emphasise that a healthy and satisfying sex life is an important part of being human.

It is not unusual for you to feel embarrassed regarding talking about sex to patients, and this could lead you to avoid eye contact, turn away from the patient, take copious notes or resort to complex jargon. You need to be aware of feelings of embarrassment, to think about your own attitudes to sex, and to become as well informed about the subject and as comfortable as possible.

Power dynamics

Keep in mind the power dynamics between yourself and your patient. For example, an adolescent boy may feel uncomfortable talking about sex to a female health professional, even though they share the same race and language.

In any situation where there are differences between the two of you, you must work harder than usual to build a trusting, open and comfortable relationship, using all the tools at your disposal (see the explanation of phase I of the core counselling skills on page 45). Remember to be non-judgemental, and try to be empathic. Assure the patient about confidentiality, and acknowledge how difficult it is for all of us to talk about sex.

How to counsel adults

There is no single correct way to begin a discussion about sex. In different cultures different norms apply. For example, in Western cultures it is more acceptable to ask direct questions than in some African cultures. In African culture, an appropriate way to approach a difficult topic such as sex is indirectly, alluding to it in non-specific terms, for example, "How is your physical relationship with your partner?"

Interestingly, patients are often much more receptive to talking about sex and sexuality than you may expect. Along with a feeling of embarrassment, many people experience an enormous sense of relief in being able to talk openly about something they have not discussed before but have thought quite a lot about.

Many adults are often not well informed about sexual anatomy. You may need to give a simple explanation of the sex organs to begin with. Use a three-dimensional model or simple illustrations, if possible.

Avoid language which is very medical and technical, and thus difficult for your patient to understand. Try to use layperson's terms as much as possible.

Issues that many patients want to learn more about include: masturbation, their own physiology, physiology of the opposite sex, what is 'normal' sexual intercourse, protection against HIV/Aids, how to talk to a partner about condoms, symptoms of STIs and how to obtain treatment.

Tips for dealing with sexual minorities

- ❑ Do not assume that your patient is heterosexual. Bisexual, lesbian and gay sexual orientations are often overlooked in medical settings. Tailor your discussion to meet the needs of your patient. And never assume sexual behaviour based on a person's appearance. Even if you think a patient is heterosexual, it is helpful to mention in a matter-of-fact way that many patients have also had same-sex sexual partners, and to ask whether this might have happened to them.
- ❑ The most helpful approach in talking to sexual minorities is one of acceptance and non-judgement. Remember that consensual, satisfying sexual behaviour, which does not interfere with a person's functioning, does not need curing.
- ❑ Ask questions that are open-ended. For example, "Do you have a partner?" is preferable to "Are you married?"
- ❑ Sexual identity and sexual behaviour are flexible. For example, a patient may identify themseves at different times of their life as heterosexual, gay and bisexual. A male patient who identifies himself as heterosexual may occasionally have sex with another man, but feel embarrassed to mention it to you.
- ❑ Be careful not to associate any particular sexual behaviour with a particular group. For example, anal penetrative sex is often associated with gay men. In fact, only a minority of gay men practise anal sex, and the largest number of practitioners of anal sex are heterosexual. So even with a heterosexual patient, male or female, it is important to ask whether they may have had anal sex.
- ❑ Many sexual minorities are concerned that they will be seen by you as disturbed just because of their sexual identities and behaviour. You will have a better professional relationship if you can assure them – truthfully – that you do not consider their sexuality to be, in and of itself, a problem.
- ❑ If you find working with sexual minorities uncomfortable, it is your responsibility to acquire more knowledge through reading or study, or to talk to a professional counsellor about your difficulties. Otherwise, you need to refer the patient to someone who is not going to be judgemental.

Tips for counselling teenagers

- It is now common for teenagers to learn about sexuality at school. However, remember that the quality of sex education given to teenagers may vary.
- Teenage boys and girls may feel embarrassment about sexual issues, but at the same time they want to find out the facts. Do not be deterred by giggling or an initial reticence to talk on their part.
- Ask a teenager to tell you about what they know. The response you get will tell you how much basic information you need to provide.
- Often teenagers are informed about the physiology and workings of the reproductive system. However, they may know little about how to negotiate relationships and how to communicate with sexual partners. Teenagers say that these skills are just as important to them as knowledge of physiology.
- Teenagers are often concerned about how normal they are, especially in terms of masturbation and sexual experience, or lack of it. Reassure them that there are many variations in sexual expression.
- Teenagers often want to learn about dating, pregnancy, masturbation, sexual orientation, oral sex, dealing with sexual abuse, protecting themselves against HIV/Aids, and where to get help with STIs.
- Remember to mention same-sex attraction and to reassure teenagers who have had these feelings that they are normal. They do not necessarily lead to a gay or lesbian orientation. However, remember too that some teenagers with feelings of same-sex attraction will grow up to be gay and lesbian. Teenagers need to be assured that the feelings are normal, in either event.
- Currently the age of consent for sex is 16 years for heterosexual sex and 19 years for homosexual sex. However, there are plans to equalise the age of consent.
- Teenagers who feel good about themselves and are able to assert themselves in the face of peer pressure are likely to delay sex until they are older. Building up their self-esteem and helping them to think about how to respond to pressure from another teenager to have sex will give them important skills to deal with peer pressure.

Talking about sex

It is often helpful to introduce the topic in words like these:

"I am going to ask some very personal questions now. We ask these questions of everyone, because we think that a person's sex life is an important aspect of health. Having sexual feelings is normal. Sex is something that can help a person feel better about themselves.

"You may be feeling embarrassed, but that's normal. Is it okay for us to carry on?

"If there are any questions you don't feel comfortable answering, feel free to tell me at any stage."

Then follow up with some general questions:

"How do you feel about your sex life? Is it satisfying for you?"

"Are you currently having sex with one or more partners? How do you feel about talking to your partner or partners about sex?"

"Do you have sex with men, women or both?"

"Do you have any concerns about sex? Tell me about them."

"Can you discuss safer sex with your partners? Would you like to discuss how to talk about safer sex?"

It is then useful to talk about more specific issues relevant to the patient, such as STIs, how to practise safer sex, birth control, etc.

Communicating effectively with children

Tips for giving information to children

- Remember that each young patient is unique. This means that there is no single approach to communicating that is correct for all children.
- The style of communication needs to be adapted to fit the age of the patient, as well as the patient's level of emotional and cognitive development. See below for some pointers on communication at different ages.
- Allow time to build a relationship with the child, using appropriate strategies, depending on the child's age. See below for more details.
- Adapt the use of language to match the language abilities of the child. Use simple vocabulary and avoid medical jargon.
- Take time to find out what the child already knows or thinks about their condition. For example, often a child thinks that getting ill is a result of being bad. So, in addition to the illness, the child takes on the burden of blaming themselves for wrongdoing. It is important to correct these myths.
- Be honest as much as possible with children. For example, do not try to hide the truth about a procedure that may cause pain. If, for example, you deny that a procedure will be painful and then it does cause pain to the child, your relationship with the child will be affected negatively. It will be more difficult to secure co-operation on the next occasion that the patient visits a clinic or hospital.
- Allow children to ask questions. Do not discount questions that sound odd or not related to the issue under discussion.
- Try wherever possible to build a relationship over time. Children often take time to develop a sense of trust, especially of an adult in unfamiliar surroundings.

Creative ways of communicating with children

Here is a range of ideas for making communicating with children easier:

- **Storytelling**. Ask the child to tell a story about an event, for example being admitted to hospital. Show them a suitable picture and ask them to tell a story about it. This strategy can provide useful feedback about the child's feelings and thoughts about a particular situation.
- **Mutual storytelling**. Get the child to tell a story. Then tell a similar story of your own, changing any negative outcome to make it more favourable. This technique can help you to pass on to the child ideas for coping.
- **Bibliotherapy**. Give the child a simple book to read about the issue, for example leukaemia. Talk to the child afterwards about what they learnt from the book. This option is useful for older children who can read well.
- **Rating game**. Ask the child to pick a face from a selection of pictures of happy and sad faces to show you how they feel. This is an easy way of finding out about emotional issues, especially with younger children.
- **Sentence completion**. Ask the child to complete a sentence that you start. For example, "The thing I am most scared of in the world is …" It helps to identify problem issues that need to be addressed.
- **'What if' questions**. To help the child to develop coping skills, you could ask them how they would cope with various concrete situations, for example "How would you cope if you had to stay in hospital?"

Talking to children of different ages

Talking to children up to 6 years of age

- Children in this age group may be very distrustful of adults they do not know.
- It is usually easier to talk to the child in the presence of a close loved one, such as a parent or guardian.
- In order to build a relationship with the child, it is helpful to get down on the floor with them and play a short game first.
- The child will not understand abstract ideas, and so everything needs to be communicated in concrete terms. Avoid metaphors that can be misinterpreted, for example "You'll get a stick in the arm" may be literally interpreted as having a piece of wood inserted.
- The child will be easily distracted by outside stimuli, so communicate with them in an environment as quiet and free from distraction as possible.
- The child needs to be given information in small chunks and it helps to repeat key messages.
- The child is likely to think that illness is a result of bad behaviour and is a punishment. At this age the child feels little control over illness and recovery.
- It will not be useful to tell a child of this age: "We have tested you for HIV and you are positive". Instead, you could tell the child "You have a special sickness". Explain further that the child may not feel ill, but needs to take special care of themselves. Then explain two very simple ways in which the child could do this, such as eating plenty of food and telling the parent if they feel unwell.

Talking to 7–11-year-olds

- Children of this age understand the world in terms of their everyday experiences: what they can see, touch and manipulate.

- It is usually possible to see the child without the parent or guardian. However, if the child is emotionally immature, they may be more comfortable with an older person present.
- One way of building a good relationship with a child of this age is to make use of storytelling or to play a game.
- The child needs to be provided with information based on concrete and practical examples.
- Children of this age want explanations for everything. They are also very concerned about bodily integrity – will something hurt? – and loss of precious possessions, like a valued and comforting toy.
- The child will appreciate being given the chance to ask questions.
- At this age the child can begin to understand the idea of infectious agents causing illness. They will be less likely to blame themselves for the illness. There is a greater sense of control over illness and recovery.
- You could tell the child in this age group who tests HIV-positive: "You have a sickness called HIV". Explain further that the child cannot make other children sick through ordinary contact. Explain three slightly more complex ways in which the child can take care of themselves, such as following a healthy diet with lots of vegetables and fruit, covering up wounds if they bleed, and taking medication properly.

Talking to teenagers

- The child's ability to understand abstract principles and to reason logically is usually fully developed by the teens, and is similar to an adult's ability.
- Teenagers can also project themselves into the future and will want to know about the long-term implications of an illness.

- In order to build a relationship, ask the teenager about their hobbies, favourite music or plans for the future.
- Children in this age group may be very distrustful of adults. It may take some time to win their trust.
- If the teenager is 14 years or older, the parent or guardian does not need to be included in information sharing, unless the teenager gives consent. (Note that in terms of changes to the Children's Act, this age limit will eventually drop to 12 years – see the section on **Obtaining informed consent** on page 74.)
- Teenagers may be able to understand information cognitively, but this does not always mean that they have the emotional capacity to deal with its implications. They may need more help with the emotional issues. They can also fluctuate between very adult behaviour and very childlike emotional responses. Remember to be empathic and non-judgemental about such behaviour.
- A teenager who tests HIV-positive could be told: "Your tests show that you are HIV-positive. How do you feel about this? Can you tell me what it means to be HIV-positive?" Check the teenager's understanding of all aspects of HIV, including how the virus affects the immune system, the difference between HIV and Aids, transmission, how the virus is not transmitted, treatment and positive lifestyle. A teen may need particular help with dating, how to negotiate safer sex and how to use a condom.

Talking to cognitively impaired patients

Tips for talking to a cognitively impaired patient

- Avoid using abstract language. Stick to concrete ways of expressing yourself to a cognitively impaired person.
- Do not treat this patient as if they were just a young child. A cognitively impaired adult needs to be treated with the respect that an adult normally gets.
- Remember that a cognitively impaired patient may have a short attention span. Give information in small, digestible chunks.
- Use active constructions and avoid passive sentence forms. Avoid negative constructions too. For example, do not say, "This medication shouldn't be taken without food". Rather say, "When you take this medication, always take it with food".
- Avoid ambiguous language that may confuse the patient.
- Draw pictures to help communicate difficult messages.
- Remember to use basic principles of counselling such as reflecting feelings (in simple ways), respect and empathy.
- Where possible, ask simple questions to check understanding.
- After talking, wait patiently for a response.
- Try not to keep the patient waiting for too long before you see them. They are likely to become tired and less able to take in new information.
- A cognitively impaired patient is more easily distracted by outside stimuli such as noise and the presence of other patients. Try to talk to them in a quiet and private setting.
- Involve family members where possible. Try to give information as much as possible with both the family member and the cognitively impaired patient together. This reduces the risk of the family member trying to get you to collude against the patient.

Pitfalls to avoid

- Talking in a loud voice as if the patient were hard of hearing.
- Talking to the patient condescendingly as if to a child.
- Giving too much information at one time.
- Offering too many options.
- Talking to the family members and ignoring the patient.

Counselling for HIV testing

Pre-test counselling

Counselling for HIV testing is different from conventional counselling, where the patient directs the process. In HIV pre-test counselling you lead by asking relevant questions and making sure that all the important issues about testing and HIV/Aids are covered. At least 20 minutes should be allocated to this process.

Patient-initiated testing

Pre-test counselling

The pre-test counselling session has two aims:

1. To educate the patient about HIV/Aids and risk reduction.
2. To help the patient decide on whether or not to do the test.

Tips for patient-initiated pre-test counselling

- ❑ Ask what made the patient decide to come forward for testing.
- ❑ Explore the patient's knowledge of HIV/Aids. Fill in the gaps.
- ❑ Talk about how the test works, including what a positive and a negative result both mean.
- ❑ Explain the window period – it can take up to three months from infection for HIV antibodies to develop.
- ❑ Talk about how to reduce the risk of contracting HIV.
- ❑ Explore how the patient will cope with a positive test result. Take time with this part of the counselling.
- ❑ Allow time for questions.

Health professional-initiated testing

Many health professionals initiate the idea of testing with a patient before the patient suggests it. This is often because you has diagnosed a condition that seems to be related to HIV, or the patient's health suggests the strong possibility that they are HIV-positive.

Pre-test counselling

The patient may not have suspected they were HIV-positive, or they may deny this possibility. So pre-test counselling may combine features of breaking bad news – "There is a possibility that you may be HIV-positive" – and persuading the patient that being tested is a good idea – "Testing will help us decide how best to treat you". Knowing the patient's status may help in making appropriate choices about patient care and treatment.

Remember that no matter how strongly you feel about HIV testing, it is still the patient's legal right to decide whether or not to be tested. The patient cannot be tested against their will.

Tips for health professional-initiated pre-test counselling

- ❑ Tell the patient what has made you think they might be HIV-positive. Do this gently but clearly.
- ❑ Introduce the advantages of being tested, especially in terms of treatment options. Knowing that treatment is readily available may be a powerful incentive to get tested.
- ❑ Explore the patient's knowledge of HIV/Aids and fill in any gaps.
- ❑ Talk about how the test works, including what positive and negative results mean.
- ❑ Explain the window period.
- ❑ Explore how the patient will cope with a positive test result.
- ❑ Explain treatment options, should the test result be positive.
- ❑ Allow time for questions.

Post-test counselling

For both health professional-initiated and patient-initiated counselling, the procedure for post-test counselling is very similar. The length of time it takes may vary from five minutes for a negative result to an hour, where the result is positive and the patient is very emotional about it.

Giving a negative result

The focus here is on encouraging the patient to stay HIV-negative. First, make sure the patient understands the result correctly. Encourage them to think about how to reduce the risk of HIV infection, through condom use. Then suggest that the patient returns for another test after the window period of three months is up.

Giving a positive result

The patient who is diagnosed HIV-positive often goes into a state of emotional shock. So the counselling session in which the news is given to the patient often has to be devoted to containing the patient – helping them to adjust to the news. The patient's emotional state makes it hard for them to take in important information that should also be given about how to live with HIV. It is helpful, where possible, to provide such information in a second session.

Tips for giving a positive result

- ❑ Give the test result calmly and allow the patient time to respond.
- ❑ Let the patient express their feelings and deal with these empathically. Remember to use counselling skills such as reflecting feelings and empathy.
- ❑ Talk about living positively with HIV (see section on **Counselling on living positively with HIV** below). Discuss treatment options where appropriate.

- ❑ Provide ideas on social support, such as talking to an HIV/Aids counsellor.
- ❑ Encourage the patient to think about disclosing their HIV-positive status, for example to their partner.
- ❑ Assess whether there is a suicide risk. Take action if the risk is high (see **Assessing suicide risk** below).
- ❑ Arrange a follow-up session where possible.

Pitfalls to avoid in pre-test and post-test counselling

- ❑ Coercing the patient into agreeing to be tested.
- ❑ Failing to talk about risk reduction in ways that the patient can relate to.
- ❑ Failing to check that the patient understands the test result.
- ❑ Not allowing time for the patient to talk about feelings in response to a positive result.
- ❑ Giving insufficient information about living positively.
- ❑ Ending a counselling session quickly because the patient says very little.

Counselling on living positively with HIV

Many patients lose hope when they test HIV-positive. They think that all that is left for them is waiting to die an agonising death. However, many people who are HIV-positive live a quality life for years. There is a lot they can do to stay healthy.

You can encourage HIV-positive patients by offering ideas on living positively. Remember to adapt your ideas to match the patient's lifestyle. For example, suggesting to an unemployed mother living in an informal settlement that she should exercise regularly is unhelpful – she probably gets enough exercise just doing her daily housework. By contrast, an office worker who spends most of their working days at a desk probably needs to be encouraged to do more exercise.

Offer a few ideas at a time. Do not overwhelm the patient by providing all these ideas at once.

Remember too that any kind of behaviour change is difficult, even when a person is feeling healthy and happy. The emotional impact of being HIV-positive makes behaviour change on the patient's part that much more difficult.

Encourage change by offering praise when the patient is able to make even small changes in the direction of living more healthily.

Tips for living positively with HIV

- ❑ Follow a healthy diet. Eat lots of fresh vegetables and fruit. Avoid too much fast food, spicy food and greasy food.
- ❑ Get lots of regular sleep.
- ❑ Exercise moderately. This can involve simple measures such as walking, playing sport and gardening.
- ❑ Cut down on smoking and alcohol if possible.
- ❑ Have regular medical check-ups.
- ❑ Take immune boosters or vitamin supplements, under medical supervision.

- ❑ Avoid re-infection by using condoms when having sex.
- ❑ Disclose your HIV status to someone you trust when you feel ready to do so.
- ❑ Talk to a counsellor if you feel depressed or sad.
- ❑ Join a support group.
- ❑ Learn as much about HIV as you can. Get informed by watching TV programmes about HIV, getting pamphlets from clinics, listening to radio programmes and asking health professionals questions about HIV.
- ❑ Get in touch with your spirituality, whether it means attending mosque, praying, joining a church choir or just enjoying nature.
- ❑ Keep a journal to write down frustrations and worries. Keep it in a safe place.
- ❑ Plan for your future.
- ❑ Live with hope; do not just plan for dying.
- ❑ Get antiretroviral treatment when you get more sick and need it.

Pitfalls to avoid

- ❑ Giving information too soon after testing.
- ❑ Giving too much information about a positive lifestyle.
- ❑ Rattling off these ideas to the patient like a shopping list.
- ❑ Not individualising counselling about a positive lifestyle.
- ❑ Expecting a patient to change their entire lifestyle overnight.

Risk reduction counselling for HIV/Aids

Research studies suggest that there are no universal messages about risk reduction that are applicable to all patients and to all situations. Generalised messages do not seem to alter patients' risk behaviours. It is more useful for you to tailor messages about risk reduction to suit the particular circumstances of the patient.

Remember to use the principles outlined in **Section A: Core communication theories**, and basic counselling principles described in **Section B: Core counselling skills**. Useful counselling skills here include empathy, non-judgement, asking open questions and summarising.

Summary of risk factors

- The most common cause of infection is through sexual transmission, and in particular **vaginal and anal penetrative sexual intercourse** without the use of a condom. Oral sex poses a lower risk.
- There is also a risk of transmission through **contact with blood**, usually through accidents.
- Another source of risk, important to remember in a southern African context, is **tattooing, initiation rites and traditional healer rituals**, including circumcision, scarification of the skin and sharing of needles or blades.
- Care-givers, usually women, who are involved in **home-based care** of HIV-positive family members, are at risk where precautions are not taken to prevent contact with the HIV-positive patient's body fluids. This risk is thought to be very low.
- The most common cause of infection for children is **mother-to-child transmission** of HIV, which occurs in the uterus during childbirth, or through breastfeeding after birth.

- There is a risk of infection for healthcare workers such as health professionals and nurses through **needle-stick injuries**, although the risk is fairly low. Post-exposure prophylaxis will reduce the risk even further.

Reducing risk for the patient

Ideas for risk reduction need to be adapted to the patient, taking account of their context.

For example, advising a woman in an abusive relationship in which she is dependent on her male partner to use a condom is probably unhelpful. In such a setting, the woman will find it almost impossible to suggest condom use without incurring further abuse. Here, the short-term goal may be to build up the woman's self-esteem and internal locus of control, so that she stops being dependent on her abusive partner. The long-term goal may be to make the woman able to assert herself in the relationship safely, or able to leave the relationship if she wishes to do so.

In the case of a male teenager who is already sexually active, for example, advising him to abstain from sex may not be the most useful strategy. Here, it may be more helpful to encourage condom use and provide easy access to condoms.

Do not assume that a patient's sexual orientation is heterosexual, and make the mistake of providing information about penile–vaginal intercourse only. Gay men and lesbians are also at risk of HIV infection but need different messages to heterosexual men and women. For example, gay men may engage in anal or oral sexual intercourse, and need information about correct condom use. Lesbians may need information about using dental dams for oral sex. Remember too that many lesbians in South Africa may have had sexual intercourse with men, have been exposed to HIV and so be at risk, or may be survivors of rape.

Example of a risk counselling session

Doctor: André, let's discuss how you can reduce your risk of getting infected with HIV. How do you feel about talking about it?

André: Well, doc, I already know the facts; I've read all about Aids.

Doctor: I'm glad you know a lot already, André. That's going to make my job easier. But do you mind if we talk anyway?

André: Sure, doc.

Doctor: The biggest risk for you is likely to be sexual transmission. HIV can be transmitted to you any time you have sex with another person – woman or man. That applies to vaginal sex, anal sex, oral sex.

André: And what about pulling out before I come? That must make it safe.

Doctor: No, André, the risk of getting HIV is there as long as you insert your penis into anyone else – as long as you don't use a condom and as long as you don't use it properly.

André: But I only have sex with women I know who are healthy.

Doctor: You can't tell from anyone's appearance who has HIV and who hasn't. Plenty of HIV-positive people look healthy.

André: So I have to use a condom every time? That's too much to ask!

Doctor: I can hear it's hard for you to think about condoms, André. But every time you don't use a condom you put yourself at risk.

André: But if I use a condom, the girl will say I must have Aids.

Doctor: How about saying, "We don't know each other's status. Let's rather protect each other by using a condom"? Would that work?

André: I can try it. But what about blood, and working with people who have HIV?

Doctor: If you help someone who has been in an accident and is bleeding, cover your hands first, even if it's just with a plastic bag. But bleeding is much lower risk for you than sex is. And ordinary contact in the workplace with anyone living with HIV, or even Aids, is no risk.

André: What else should I worry about?

Doctor: Don't share razors or blades with anyone else. If you get tattooed, make sure the person doing the tattooing uses proper hygienic methods.

André: Uh-huh.

Doctor: Let's go back again to condoms. Tell me what you know about using them properly.

André: You've got to store them properly – not in a trouser pocket or in a car. Also, check the expiry date. Make sure to open them carefully and not damage them.

Doctor: That's good. And you need to use proper lubricant – do you know what that is?

André: Any sort of cream.

Doctor: No, it has to be water-based lubricant, like KY gel. If you use an oil-based lubricant like hand cream, it can make the condom tear.

André: Okay.

Doctor: Any more questions?

André: No, doc, I think I've got it now.

Doctor: Next time you come, let's talk again and see how you're doing with protecting yourself.

Tips for talking about condoms

- Most adults have heard about condoms but may not know how to use them.
- There are many myths about condoms, such as they spread HIV, they can get stuck in a woman. Ask the patient what they believe about condoms and challenge these myths if they are mentioned.
- For many adults the biggest difficulty is how to introduce the idea of condoms to their partner.
- It can be helpful to practise with the patient what they can say to the partner about introducing condoms to the relationship.
- Learning to use condoms correctly and getting used to them takes time.
- Remember also to advise about correct storage, checking of the expiry date, use of water-based lubricant only and correct disposal.
- Don't give up if the patient does not use a condom after the first time they are mentioned. It may take time for the patient to get accustomed to the idea.

Tips for HIV harm reduction

- Ask about the patient's background and sexual history, where appropriate.
- Check on their basic knowledge of HIV/Aids.
- Work out the main risk factors for the patient.
- Counsel about the most relevant methods of risk reduction.
- If you talk about condoms, give details about how to use them too.
- Give risk reduction messages on more than one occasion, where possible.
- Ask the patient what they think is helpful in terms of risk reduction.

Pitfalls to avoid

- Giving vague information about risk reduction.
- Moralising about HIV/Aids.
- Not adjusting ideas about risk reduction to suit the needs of the patient.
- Discouraging the patient from asking questions.

Counselling on taking antiretroviral medication

As the Aids pandemic worsens, more and more people in South Africa will need to be given antiretroviral treatment (ART). In order for the treatment to work, a patient needs to take at least 19 out of every 20 doses correctly. This means taking the correct combination of medication, in the correct dose, at the correct time.

Getting patients to adhere to treatment means more than merely telling them when and how to take their medicine. As with any other form of behaviour change, information provision alone does not make patients take their medication (see **Section A: Core communication skills**). Getting patients to adhere also involves building a clear motivation for the behaviour change, developing new skills, integrating the new behaviour into their lifestyle, and addressing obstacles to the new behaviour.

Increasingly, the responsibility of counselling patients on ART does not fall just on the counsellor or nurse. Instead, every member of the health care team can help to reinforce messages about taking the treatment correctly by talking informally to the patient at every opportunity that there is for health professional–patient contact.

Tips for talking to a patient about ART adherence

- ❑ Remember that taking any long-term treatment is a challenge for any patient, let alone a patient having to learn to live with an HIV-positive status.
- ❑ Develop a teamwork approach to making the medication work: this is about you, the nurse, dietician, pharmacist, counsellor and patient all working together to make taking medication easier.

- Prepare the patient well in advance. Discuss all the implications of ART, including the importance of adherence, the dangers of non-adherence, possible side-effects and the benefits of the medication.
- Talk about any fears and worries the patient may have.
- Describe the dangers of non-adherence – that the patient may develop resistance to the medication.
- Tell the patient what side-effects to look out for, and what action to take if the side-effects develop. Use simple, non-medical language.
- Help the patient to develop a strong motivation for taking ART. Ask them: "How could you benefit from getting some extra years of quality life?"
- Think together of some useful ideas that can assist the patient in taking treatment more easily (see the ideas for making adherence easier below).
- Allow time for the patient to ask questions.
- Once the patient has started treatment, offer plenty of encouragement.
- Where possible, encourage the patient to attend a support group.
- Offer counselling on return visits to reinforce messages about adherence.
- If problems develop later with regard to adherence, do not blame the patient. Instead, try to problem-solve together.
- Celebrate successful adherence – six months on treatment, then one year on treatment are major reasons for celebration!

Here are some ideas for making adherence easier:

- Keeping medication in a place where it is visible, for example with the toothbrush or next to the kettle.
- Using a portable pillbox to carry medication at all times, which is especially useful when the patient moves around a lot.

- Recording on a wallchart, calendar or diary every time treatment is taken.
- Setting a regular reminder message on the patient's cellphone.
- Using cellphone SMSs to remind the patient.
- Having a buddy-on-treatment to support the patient.
- Using a family member to remind the patient.
- Encouraging the patient to join a support group.
- Using an alarm clock or watch alarm to help remind the patient.
- Associating taking treatment with certain regular radio or TV programmes.

Pitfalls to avoid

- Just giving information.
- Giving all the information at once.
- Forgetting the challenges of living with HIV.
- Giving counselling only at the beginning of treatment.
- Forgetting that the patient has the right to decide whether or not to take treatment.

Example of an antiretroviral treatment (ART) adherence counselling session

Patient: Morning, Sister. I've come for my monthly visit.

Nurse: Morning, Mary. It's two months now since you began ART. How are you doing?

Patient: Fine thanks, Sister. It's not easy, but I'm managing.

Nurse: Do you want to tell me a bit about how it's been going? [Open-ended question]

[Less useful question: Have you been taking your medication all the time?]

Patient: Well, I've been taking my medication as I'm supposed to ... I just feel very tired all the time and then I want to sleep. I can't cook and clean like before. I'm so tired when I wake up that I'm scared that I'll sleep through my morning dose.

Nurse: It sounds like it's been difficult for you. Do you think your tiredness could be a side-effect of the medication?

[Less useful response: It's very important that you don't miss any doses. You know that you have to take your medication at the same time every day!]

Patient: Yes, I think it is. The counsellor told me that I might feel like this. He also said that I might get diarrhoea from the AZT/3TC.

Nurse: Has knowing this made it any easier to cope with – knowing that what you're experiencing is common?

[Less useful response: I'm sure it will go away soon. Just keep taking your medication.]

Patient: Yes, I guess it has. I probably would have got a fright if I hadn't expected it. I bought bananas, rice and apple-sauce for the diarrhoea, just in case. So I was prepared.

Nurse: It sounds like you're being responsible, Mary. So you're eating bananas, rice, apple-sauce and toast?

Patient: (Laughs) Yes! But Sister… some days I'm tempted not to take my medication. I don't like the way it's making me feel.

Nurse: Perhaps you have days when you wonder if this is worth it. Maybe the side-effects make you feel worse than the HIV was making you feel before you started treatment?

[Less useful response: You know that it's really important to keep persisting. Everyone feels that way.]

Patient: Yes. (Starts crying) I know … that … it's really important for me to take the drugs every day, and I'm worried … that I'll forget and then the drugs won't work any more and I'll get sick and die. There'll be nothing left for me.

Nurse: It sounds like you feel scared. I can see that you know how important it is to take your medication, but it seems like you're putting a lot of pressure on yourself too. Would you like to talk about how you can manage these side-effects more easily?

[Less useful response: You have to pull yourself together, otherwise you'll make yourself sicker than you are now. Do you want that?]

Patient: Yes, please. I really need to see if there are things that will help me to get through this.

Containing traumatised patients

A common occurrence in a medical setting is a patient suffering from some form of psychological trauma. It is helpful to know the symptoms of trauma, and to have some understanding of how to help the patient to feel contained and supported. Moreover, it is important to know where patients who suffer more severely from post-traumatic stress disorder (PTSD) may be referred for help.

Remember to use the counselling skills of empathy and unconditional acceptance to help the patient to tell their story. Also make use of appropriate open-ended questions.

Causes

A trauma reaction can be triggered by any of the following situations:

- ❑ Being a victim of crime, including robbery, hijacking, being held up at gunpoint, shooting, housebreaking and rape.
- ❑ Witnessing another person being the victim of crime.
- ❑ Being involved in a vehicle accident, fire, flood or any other natural disaster.
- ❑ Witnessing other people being hurt in an accident.
- ❑ Witnessing someone killing someone else, or committing suicide.
- ❑ Receiving a diagnosis of being HIV-positive.
- ❑ Receiving a diagnosis of having a terminal or life-threatening illness.

Recognising the symptoms

The symptoms that a patient may show in reaction to trauma vary a great deal, but can include any of the following:

- ...n the form of sweaty palms, increased heart- ... trembling.
- Being very emotional – tearful, sad or angry – or in a state of shock.
- Feeling generally edgy and nervous.
- An exaggerated startle response, for example the patient getting a fright when someone comes up behind them.
- Strong fear of the original situation.
- Fear of any other situation resembling it, or of anyone resembling the perpetrator.
- Poor concentration.
- Change in libido.
- Change in eating patterns.
- Inability to plan appropriately or to think ahead.
- Getting into more conflict than usual with people in the immediate environment, including family members and friends.
- Sleeping poorly at night, sleeping more than normal, or being woken by nightmares.

How to respond

During the period immediately after the traumatic event has occurred, the patient is most likely to be in a state of shock. They may also experience a roller-coaster of emotions, including anxiety, anger, fear, sadness, terror and even thoughts of suicide. What the patient needs most in this period is not counselling but just assistance in feeling safe and contained.

Tips for responding within 24 hours of the trauma

- Give the patient a cup of tea or some other comforting beverage while you talk to them, in private if possible.
- If the patient wants to talk about their experience, allow them to do so. But do not turn the talk into a formal counselling session, as the trauma will be too recent for the patient to benefit from trying to process it.

- Tell the patient what to expect in the next few days – see the list of symptoms above.
- Make sure that the patient is shielded from having to talk to lots of curious bystanders about their experience, unless they wish to do so.
- If the patient has family members or friends who can be supportive, encourage these people to offer support. Tell the family members about the symptoms of trauma the patient might experience.
- Some traumatised people prefer not to be left alone during this period. Check with the patient what they would find most supportive.
- Let the patient decide how much or how little they wish to discuss about the experience. Some patients benefit from talking repeatedly to others, telling their story in great detail; others prefer to be left alone to process the experience by themselves.

Where possible, make a follow-up appointment with the patient. Allow 48 hours to pass before giving counselling to the person who has been traumatised. This period gives the patient sufficient time to move out of the state of shock and to begin to process the experience.

Tips for counselling after 48 hours has passed

- Encourage the patient to talk in detail about the traumatic event, recalling as much of the experience as they feel comfortable with.
- Ask them to begin by recalling what was happening before the trauma occurred, then to describe the trauma, and finally to recall what they thought and how they reacted afterwards.
- If the patient starts to feel very anxious about recalling the traumatic event, suggest they remember the event as if they were standing outside it and watching it happen on TV. So, for example, they can say, "I saw on TV a man walking down the street and then someone pulled out

a gun and pointed it at him ..." This method may seem artificial but it establishes a clear and safe distance from the event.

- Ask the patient how they responded to the trauma emotionally. Normalise their reaction.
- Describe the symptoms that the patient might expect to have. However, point out that every traumatised person reacts differently, and there is no right or wrong response.
- Ask how the patient usually copes with stress. Encourage the patient to use an adaptive response such as talking to another person, doing exercise and writing down their feelings. Suggest appropriate responses if the patient has no ideas.
- Tell the patient that if the symptoms worsen or persist for more than a month, they should consider seeking more formal help.
- Make the patient aware of referral options such as trauma counselling services, for example, Lifeline (whose 24-hour crisis number is 0861 322 322) and the Centre for the Study of Violence and Reconciliation (CSVR) in Johannesburg (whose contact number is 011 403 5102/3).

Pitfalls to avoid

- Just offering tea and sympathy.
- Failing to normalise emotional reactions.
- Offering trauma counselling immediately after the trauma.

Recognising the risk of suicide

It is important to look out for key signs that a person may be at risk for committing suicide.

Key signs of suicide risk

- ❑ The patient has a clear plan for killing themselves – this is the highest risk factor.
- ❑ The patient has the means to carry out such a plan.
- ❑ The patient has attempted suicide before.
- ❑ The patient is an adolescent or is elderly – risk is highest in these two groups.
- ❑ The patient abuses alcohol or another harmful substance.
- ❑ The patient has a psychiatric disorder or a severe physical illness.
- ❑ The patient expresses feelings of hopelessness and thinks things will never get better.
- ❑ The patient is agitated and/or aggressive.

If any of these key signs are present, consider seriously the possibility that the patient may be suicidal. If the first factor is present, or any two other factors are present, consider the risk as extremely serious.

Moreover, you need to be aware of the symptoms of depression, which can also be present in a suicidal patient. These include depressed mood, changes in appetite, changes in sleep pattern, low energy, reduced pleasure in life, withdrawal, poor concentration and feelings of worthlessness.

Assessing suicide risk

If you think the patient may be at risk for suicide, it is important to talk to them about it. Do not be afraid that talking about suicide will prompt the patient to carry out the plans. On the contrary, the patient is more likely to feel relieved that the issue has been brought out into the open, and that someone is prepared to offer help.

You should ask questions about:

- how the patient is feeling currently
- whether the patient has thought about suicide, and, if so, whether they have a plan to carry it out
- whether suicide has ever been considered or attempted previously
- whether the patient uses alcohol or drugs and, if so, how much.

If you decide that there is a risk of suicide, you should ask further questions about the patient's support system. There is a greater risk in cases where the support system is poor or non-existent.

Responding to a suicidal patient

Low risk

If you decide that the risk is low, it is still helpful to think of providing support to the patient. It may be useful to talk to the patient about who they turn to for support regarding problems, and to encourage the patient to do so now. You may also make the patient aware of resources in the community, for example a church group or a support group. Finally, you may refer the patient to a lay counsellor or to a professional who can offer further counselling, such as a psychologist or social worker.

High risk

If you decide after talking to patient that the risk is high, you must take further action. The first step is for you to decide on one of the following courses of action:

- Refer the patient to psychiatric services. Make sure they are seen the same day.

- ❑ Get the patient admitted immediately to a ward and get them sedated.
- ❑ If the patient refuses to do either of these willingly and the risk is high, they may need to be certified as an involuntary patient.

The patient should not be referred for help and then sent home because they cannot be seen by a psychiatrist or psychiatric services. This is extremely risky and may allow the patient to carry out the suicidal plan. If all else fails, get the patient seen by the casualty department.

In treating the patient it is usually better to err on the side of caution. Most patients who succeed in committing suicide have given warning of their intention to do so. Remember too that an unsuccessful attempt, or attempts, in the past does not mean the patient may not now succeed in killing themselves. Talk carefully to every patient who is suicidal before making a decision on correct management.

Example of an interview with a suicidal patient

Sister: Thandi, it sounds as if things have been going badly for you in the last two months since you were told you have breast cancer. I know this is sometimes hard to talk about. But can I ask you how you are feeling now?

Thandi: (sighs and says nothing)

Sister: It looks as if you feel really sad and hopeless, like you think there is no way to carry on.

Thandi: Yes, sister.

Sister: This may sound strange, but have you ever thought of killing yourself?

Thandi: Yes, I do think about it sometimes.

Sister: Thandi, can I ask, how often have you thought of it in the past month?

Thandi: Almost every day.

Sister: Can I ask you some more questions? (*Thandi nods*) How often do you drink alcohol? How much do you drink per week?

Thandi: No, maybe two beers on a weekend. That's the only time.

Sister: And do you take anything else? Like dagga or any other pills that we haven't prescribed for you?

Thandi: No, sister. (*cries softly*)

Sister: Just because life gets too much doesn't mean you are a bad person, Thandi. Sometimes all those demands feel like a heavy load.

Thandi: Maybe it will be better for my children if I am not there. I'm not a good mother.

Sister: You're feeling like you can't cope now, but I'll make sure you get some help. We can help you manage better. Let's give it a try.

Thandi: (*nods*)

Sister: The first thing is that I want you to see a psychiatrist. He's a special doctor who talks to people who feel they aren't coping. He'll speak to you and decide whether you need to be admitted to hospital – just to give you a break from your family. And also, he'll see whether you need special pills to help you feel better. Then, we'll see if there is someone for you to talk to about your problems. Any questions you want to ask me?

Thandi: No, sister.

Sister: So, I'll write a letter for you to take along to see him. I'll show you where to go now.

Tips for dealing with a suicidal patient

- Be aware of the risk factors that suggest suicide.
- Treat every patient who has any sign of being suicidal as potentially at risk.
- Ask the patient directly about thoughts or plans of suicide.
- Check on the patient's support system and encourage them to make use of it.
- If the risk of suicide is high, consider hospitalisation.
- If a patient at high risk will not accept hospitalisation, get them certified.

Pitfalls to avoid

- Ignoring warning signs of suicide.
- Asking vague and indirect questions.
- Not intervening for fear of being wrong.

Counselling patients on treatment options

In medical settings, patients often need help from health professionals to make decisions about medical treatment. For example:

- A married couple may need to decide which option to choose to treat infertility.
- A young gay man may need to make a decision about whether or not to be tested for HIV, after having a sexual encounter with an HIV-positive man in which a condom broke.
- A 30-year-old woman and her fiancé may be faced with deciding whether or not the woman should undergo facial reconstructive surgery after she has experienced a serious injury in a car accident.
- A teenage girl may need to make up her mind regarding whether or not to terminate her pregnancy.
- A 65-year-old man with terminal liver cancer may be faced with a decision, in consultation with his children, as to whether or not he should have the cancer treated.

Remember that no decision about treatment options is a purely rational, medical decision. The decision needs to take into account the patient's values, life circumstances, financial resources and personal preferences.

Use the counselling principles outlined in **Section B: Core counselling skills**, including empathy, asking open-ended questions, clarifying and being sensitive to cultural differences.

Also see the section on **Obtaining informed consent** (page 74) for details about the age of consent for different procedures.

Tips for counselling about treatment options

- It may be helpful to think first of who needs to be given information in order to make an informed decision. Do family members need to be included? If you are not sure, ask the patient.
- Make sure that wherever possible, enough time is set aside to discuss the options fully. This is especially important in the case of life-threatening conditions.
- Start by asking the patient (and their family, if they are included) what they know about the particular disease or condition. This will allow you to work out how much information you need to communicate.
- Describe the disease or condition using non-clinical language as much as possible. Avoid medical jargon.
- List in simple terms the options for treatment. It may be useful to write these down for the patient, if they are literate. Pictures or simple diagrams may also help to explain the options.
- Describe the advantages and disadvantages of each treatment option.
- Check that the patient and the family members have understood what has been spoken about.
- Give an opportunity for the patient and relatives to ask questions.
- Where feasible, give the patient and the relatives educational materials to take way with them.
- If possible, allow the patient some time to think about the treatment options before having to return and report their decision.

Pitfalls to avoid

- Using difficult medical jargon.
- Failing to acknowledge feelings about treatment choices.
- Rushing the discussion.
- Pressurising the patient to make a particular decision.

Genetic counselling

Genetic counselling is necessary when a woman decides to have a baby and she wants to look at the risk of passing on genetic diseases or disorders to the child. Genetic counselling will help the woman, with or without the involvement of her partner, to assess the risks and to make an informed decision about continuing with the pregnancy.

Genetic counselling is the process of:

- taking and evaluating the family history and medical records for both parents
- ordering appropriate genetic tests
- evaluating the results of this investigation
- helping the woman – and, where appropriate, her partner too – to understand the implications of the genetic inheritance and decide what to do next.

Genetic counselling is a specialist skill. It is often carried out by doctors and other professionals with specialist knowledge of genetics. However, it may sometimes be necessary for non-specialist health professionals to help patients to understand what they have been told in genetic counselling and to reinforce the messages they have already received.

Many of the counselling skills outlined in this and the preceding sections may be useful to use here, including empathy, being sensitive to cultural differences, breaking bad news and dealing with loss.

Who should see a genetic counsellor?

A mother-to-be should be advised to have genetic counselling if:

- she is 35 years of age or older
- she has had two or more miscarriages, or babies that died during infancy

- either parent already has children with an inherited disease or birth defect
- either parent or a close relative has an inherited disease or birth defect
- the parents are concerned about birth defects that occur in their racial or ethnic group frequently, such as couples of central or eastern European Jewish descent with the risk of Tay-Sachs disease.

Preparing for the counselling session

Before doing any genetic counselling, the pregnant woman – and her partner, where possible – needs to be told what genetic counselling means and how it works. The woman's informed consent needs to be obtained (see **Obtaining informed consent** on page 74 for more details).

A full genetic history of both parents and their families needs to be taken. A careful physical examination of the mother and various biological tests need to be carried out in order to gather data about risk. This is best done by a genetic specialist.

The tips below pertain to counselling a pregnant woman who does not wish to involve her partner. Note, however, that the same principles apply when both parents are given counselling. Always suggest that the patient brings along a support person to the counselling session, be it her partner, a friend or another family member.

Tips for genetic counselling

- Remember that most patients who receive genetic counselling feel very anxious about the possibility of having to make a difficult decision about the pregnancy. Be empathic and reflect the patient's feelings.
- Assess the patient's coping skills. Will she be able to cope with bad news? Does she have emotional support?

- Provide the information in small, manageable chunks. As you proceed, ask questions to check her understanding.
- In talking about risk, avoid the mathematical language of probability that is confusing for most people. Rather than talk about the risk of a particular syndrome being, for example, 1 in 10, explain that out of every ten mothers in this situation, one will have a baby with the particular syndrome.
- Then allow the patient to express her immediate response to the information she has been given about the risks.
- List the choices that the patient has, and help her to think of the advantages and disadvantages of each choice.
- Avoid being judgemental or directive about the choice you think should be made.
- You may offer the patient the option of talking to other patients who have had experience of the particular genetic syndrome. There are support groups focusing on Down's syndrome, Huntingdon's syndrome, etc. which you could make use of. Such contact may help the patient to make a more informed decision.
- Genetic counselling often arouses anxiety in the patient about 'playing God' with the life of the unborn child. This often links to the patient's religious beliefs. Ask the patient what her beliefs are, and how they might affect the decision she makes.
- Remember that when a patient chooses termination of the pregnancy, she will need counselling to deal with the sense of loss and grieving (see below).
- Allow the patient to express in her own words her understanding of the discussion.
- Wherever possible, allow the patient time to go away and think before having to make a decision.
- If the genetic issues are too complex for you to understand, refer the patient formally to a genetic counsellor.

Pitfalls to avoid

- Using excessive medical jargon.
- Being overly pessimistic.
- Providing confusing information to the patient.
- Not giving the patient time to process the information.

Loss and grieving

Many current Western ideas about loss and grieving are based on the work of Dr Elisabeth Kübler-Ross, a Swiss medical doctor who worked extensively in hospital settings with people suffering from terminal illness. Based on her experience, Dr Kübler-Ross describes five basic stages of loss. These stages are not just applicable to people faced with terminal illness or death, they also occur with any individual faced with any form of loss, such as losing a loved one, losing a job, facing a change in health and testing HIV-positive.

The five stages are: denial, anger, bargaining, depression and acceptance. It is important to remember that these stages do not occur in a fixed, linear order and may be experienced simultaneously. A patient who is experiencing loss may start in the denial stage and then move to depression, and then back to anger. Another patient may never move out of the denial stage. Other patients may move backwards and forwards between several stages. All these possibilities are normal.

Notes on grieving the loss of a person

- Grieving is a normal and natural process.
- Modern life does not allow many people to grieve naturally.
- A grieving patient often needs to talk repeatedly about the person they have lost.
- A patient may shift back and forth between coping/engaging with the world, and withdrawing/becoming very emotional. This is a normal process.
- There is no correct period of time for the grieving process. Depending on the importance of the loss, it may take between 6 and 18 months.

Tips on dealing with loss and grieving

- ❑ Recognise the stage of loss or grieving which the patient is in.
- ❑ Accept the stage the patient is in.
- ❑ Reflect the patient's feelings accurately and empathically.
- ❑ Give the patient clear and practical support.
- ❑ Let the patient talk if they wish to do so. Allow the patient also to choose the option of remaining silent.
- ❑ Often just talking, sometimes about the same issue a number of times, is helpful in itself.
- ❑ Where the patient's grieving is having a major effect on their daily functioning, consider referring them for supportive counselling.
- ❑ Open communication with children is important. Concepts, however, need to be presented in an age-appropriate manner. The finality of death only becomes more completely understood around the age of 9–10 years. Younger children believe that death is separation. Between 5 and 10 years there comes the gradual recognition that death cannot be reversed.

Pitfalls to avoid

- ❑ Retaliating in an attacking way when the patient gets angry.
- ❑ Trying to cheer the patient up.
- ❑ Giving unrealistic hope.
- ❑ Giving up on the patient and simply abandoning them.

This quotation may be helpful in encouraging you to talk to patients who experience loss:

"Slowly, I learn about the importance of powerlessness. I experience it in my own life and live with it in my work. The secret is not to be afraid of it – not to run away. The dying know we are not God. All they ask is that we do not desert them."

Sheila Cassidy, a British hospice doctor, in her memoir *Sharing the Darkness*.

Counselling a patient about loss

The doctor arrives at the bedside of Sarah. Her baby was premature and taken to neonatal ICU immediately after the birth. The baby has died.

Doctor: Sarah, I'm Dr Pemba and I was the doctor who delivered your baby. I need to talk with you about your baby – please come with me to the room next door where we can talk privately.

Sarah: Is something wrong with my baby?

Doctor: Well, let's go to the room and talk.

They arrive in the room and sit down.

Doctor: Sarah, I have to tell you about your baby. As you know it was six weeks premature and very tiny. We did everything we could to save it, but I'm afraid your baby was too weak and it has died.

Sarah looks at the doctor, stunned, and then breaks into a howl of pain. This soon becomes intense sobbing. The doctor sits and waits – leans forward and waits for a while in compassionate silence.

Doctor: Sarah, this is a big shock for you.

Sarah carries on crying. The doctor sits next to her and touches her on her shoulder.

Doctor: This is a very hard thing to hear.

Sarah: But what happened?

Doctor: Well, it's hard to say exactly. It looks like the baby was just too small and its lungs and heart were not properly developed.

Sarah starts crying again and the doctor waits patiently.

Sarah: (hesitantly) This was my first baby – we wanted him so much.

Doctor: (nods) He was very precious to you.

Sarah: Yes. My husband and I had planned everything and we had given him a name already.

Doctor: So you were really looking forward to this new person in your life – what name had you given him?

Sarah: Simon. (starts crying again)

Doctor: Sarah, I can see it's really sore for you. One moment everything looked hopeful and now all that hope has gone.

Sarah: (wails) Oh God, what am I going to do?

Doctor: Is there someone we should contact for you to come and be here with you?

Sarah: My husband.

Doctor: We can make a call from my office – would you like to speak to him or do you want me to?

Sarah: I can't speak to him …

Doctor: That's fine, I'll do that – what would you like me to tell him?

Sarah: Just say he must come to see me, please, and when he comes I'll tell him.

Sarah starts crying again.

Sarah: (half angry, half tearful) It's not fair, this was supposed to be the start of our new family. Why didn't you save him? Why? Oh God!

Doctor: You know we really tried hard – we hate losing any baby like this. But unfortunately Simon was just too weak. (pauses and leans forward) It isn't fair to lose a baby like this.

Sarah sits quietly in numb silence.

Doctor: Sarah, this has been a big shock for you and when you feel ready you may want to talk to a counsellor or a minister. Now I'm going to go and make that phone call to your husband. I'll ask Sister to bring you a cup of tea. Is that okay? Is there anything else you need right now?

References

Aids Law Project. 2005. 'HIV testing and informed consent.' Accessed at www.alp.co.za (30 September 2005).

Brouard, P. 2002. *HIV/Aids counselling course manual*. Pretoria: Centre for the Study of Aids, University of Pretoria.

Cassidy, S. 1992. *Sharing the darkness, the spirituality of caring*. Orbis Books.

Cave, A. 1996. *Basic counselling skills course*. Hillbrow, Johannesburg: Community Aids Centre.

Constitution of the Republic of South Africa. 1996. Accessed at www.polity.org.za (30 September 2005).

Dallaire, L. and Huret, J.P. 2005. 'Genetics and cytogenetics.' Accessed at www.infobiogen.fr (11 September 2005).

Doyle, D.; Hanks, G. and Cherny, N. (eds). 2005. *The Oxford textbook of palliative medicine*. Third edition. Oxford: Oxford University Press.

Egan, G. 1998. *The skilled helper: A problem-management approach to helping*. Sixth edition. Pacific Grove: Brooks Cole.

Frierson, R.L.; Melikian, M. and Wadman, P.C. 2002. 'Principles of suicide risk assessment.' *Postgraduate Medicine*, 112 (3), 65–71.

Hamerdinger, S. and Karlin, B. 2005. 'Therapy using interpreters: Questions on the use of interpreters in therapeutic settings for monolingual therapists.' Accessed at www.dhs.state.il.us (29 September 2005).

Hamilton, R. 2005. *A basic 5-day counselling and VCT training course: Facilitator's manual*. Johannesburg: Aurum Health Research.

McQuoid-Mason, D. 2006. The National Health Act and refusal of consent to health services by children. *SAMJ*, 96 (6).

National Health Service. 2005. 'Giving up smoking: Understand your habit.' Accessed at www.givingupsmoking.co.uk (2 October 2005).

Twycross, R. 2003. *Introducing palliative care*. Calicut, India: Institute of Palliative Medicine.

UNAIDS. 1999. *Sexual behaviour change for HIV: Where have theories taken us?* Geneva: UNAIDS.

Van Dyk, A. 2005. *HIV/Aids care and counselling: A multidisciplinary approach*. Third edition. Cape Town: Maskew Miller Longman.

Resources

Alcoholism

Alcoholics Anonymous
Johannesburg
011 452 9907
Cape Town
021 592 5047
East Rand
011 421 1534
Pretoria
012 322 6047
Van der Bijlpark
016 455 2986
Durban
031 301 4959
Port Elizabeth
041 367 3637
East London
043 741 3865

Domestic Violence

Nicro, Cape Town - 021 422 1690
Women's Help Line - 080 015 0150
POWA (People Opposing *Woman Abuse*),
Johannesburg - 011 642 4345
Johannesburg - 011 933 2333
Stop Women Abuse - 080 015 0150

Allergy and Asthma

Allergy and Asthma Network
www.aanma.org
Allergy Society of SA, Cape Town - 021 447 9019

Anxiety Disorders
Depression and Anxiety Support Group
www.anxiety.org
080 011 8392

Child Abuse
Childline National Number - 086 132 2322
Child Emergency - 080 012 3321
Child Protection Unit of South African Police,
Cape Town
021 376 3030
021 592 2601
Durban
031 307 7000
080 011 1213

Drug Addiction
Nar-Anon Helpline - 088 129 6791
Narcotics Anonymous - 088 130 0327

Epilepsy
SA National Epilepsy League, Cape Town
021 447 3014

HIV/Aids
Napwa, Cape Town - 021 424 1106
Aids Help Line - 080 001 2322

Lifeline
24-hour crisis number - 0861 322 322
www.lifeline.org.za

National Council against Smoking
PO Box 1242, Houghton 2041
www.againstsmoking.org
Booklets currently available in English and isiZulu

Rape and Violence
Rape Crisis, Cape Town - 021 447 1467
The Triangle Project for Gay and Lesbian Rape Victims,
Cape Town - 021 442 2500
Lifeline Rape Counselling, Pretoria - 012 342 2222
Lifeline Rape Counselling (Zulu-speaking), Durban - 031 303 1344
Lifeline Rape Counselling, East London - 043 722 2000
Lifeline Rape Counselling, Port Elizabeth - 041 585 8565
Rape Crisis, Bloemfontein - 051 444 6143

The Elderly
Heal (Halt Elder Abuse Line) - 080 000 3081

Trauma Counselling Services
Trauma Clinic Counselling Network,
Cape Town - 021 683 7603

Trauma Research
Centre for the Study of Violence and Reconciliation
011 403 5102/3
www.csvr.org.za